Are You Helping Your Body Live?

Effective Ways for a Healthier Lifestyle

Runae L. Gary

Wasteland Press
Shelbyville, KY USA
www.wastelandpress.net

Are You Helping Your Body Live?
Effective Ways for a Healthier Lifestyle
by Runae L. Gary

First Printing – October 2010
ISBN: 978-1-60047-485-9

All Scripture quotations are from the
King James Version of the Holy Bible.

Printed in the U.S.A.

This book is dedicated to anyone who is struggling with any type of health challenge. It is my hope that you will find something in this book to help you, or someone you know, overcome whatever negative health issue you, or they, may be facing.

It is also dedicated to my Lord and Savior, Jesus Christ, for planting a sincere desire and passion in my heart to do what I can to help all people live a longer and much healthier life. I thank Him for allowing me to be used as one of the many vehicles on this earth to help educate people in this area. Finally, I thank Him for the several things that were revealed to me to overcome some health issues that I personally faced, and can now pass those successes on to others.

DISCLAIMER

This book, *Are You Helping Your Body Live? Effective Ways for a Healthier Lifestyle*, is not intended to diagnose or prescribe any treatment for any medical condition. It is not intended to make any claims to prevent, diagnose, treat, or cure any medical or health-related conditions.

This book contains the ideas, opinions and experiences of its author and is intended solely to provide helpful information based on those ideas, opinions and experiences of its author.

The reader should consult his or her medical health care provider or other medical professionals before incorporating any of the suggestions in this book.

The author and publisher specifically disclaim all responsibility for any liability, loss, or risk, personal or otherwise, that is incurred as a consequence (directly or indirectly) of the use and application of any of the contents of this book.

A Special Expression of Love & Thanks!

To my husband, Phillip Gary, Jr., for all your love, support and ongoing encouragement.

To my parents, Elder Rudolph Perry, Sr. & Mattie M. Perry, for being such all-around great parents and genuine examples of a healthy marriage and true holy matrimony.

To my son, Paul G. Favors, Jr., for never hesitating to share your God-given wisdom and knowledge and for being such an inspiration to me and so many others.

To my daughter-in-law, LaTasha — "Tasha" — for bringing such joy into Paul's life, which in turn brings joy into mine.

To my brother, Jeffery S. Perry, and cousin, Alfretta — "Fretta" — Miller, for all of your assistance.

To my (play) adopted daughter, Tyanna Motley, for your continued motivation in helping me to complete this assignment.

To Pastors Kenneth and Lynette Hagin, and Pastor Rick (Cindy) Fern, for having enough confidence in me, and allowing me to share my passion, by leading a Health and Wellness group during my tenure at RHEMA Bible Training Center (2006-2008), Broken Arrow, Oklahoma.

To all the health and wellness advocates, past, present and future, for all of their efforts in promoting healthier lifestyles.

And, to all the other special people in my life—you know who you are!

Table of Contents

Introduction

A young child is diagnosed with cancer. An overweight eighteen-year-old dies of a heart attack. A twenty-six-year-old has a heart attack. A thirty-three-year-old dies from congestive heart failure. A stroke attacks a fourteen-year-old. A four-year-old has severe hypertension. A two-year-old is diagnosed with high cholesterol, and a six-year-old with diabetes, and the list goes on and on. I wish that these cases were not true, but the fact of the matter is that they are. It appears as if more people are dying or being attacked with sicknesses and diseases, as well as other health problems, at much younger ages now than ever before. We could blame this on several things, but in reality, many of these premature deaths, illnesses and health problems could be avoided just by making some simple lifestyle changes.

This book is written to help individuals of all ages gain knowledge on what they can do to live longer and much healthier lives. Let's face it, who likes or wants to be sick? Who enjoys feeling the pain, hurt and suffering that come with many sicknesses and diseases? What about the family members and the caretakers who can feel so helpless as they sit back and watch a loved one suffer with pain? There are many people who lay on their deathbeds wishing they had taken better care of their bodies when they had the chance to do so. Some of these people are given another opportunity at life and are able to get up off of their sick beds, while others do not get that chance. They die either never knowing what they could have done to take better care of their bodies, or they die knowing what they could have done, never doing it, and finding themselves not having another chance at life.

Let me make this clear up front. I am not a doctor, nurse, dietitian or any of the many trained medical field professionals. I am just a person who has a sincere desire and a passion to do whatever I can to help as many people as I can live longer, healthier lives. The information that I share in this book is based strictly on my own personal experiences and findings. It is being written based on my knowledge and understanding of its contents at the time of this writing. It contains things that I have found to help me, and others as well, and would like to pass on to whoever wishes to read what I have to share.

I have been asked by several people to help them with their personal challenges as related to their health, and many have been helped by my advice. Oftentimes they are people I know. Through this book, however, I hope to reach out to individuals who I don't know, who I may not otherwise reach, and/or who can be helped in some way by the information contained herein.

Personally, I am one who is tired of seeing people get sick, suffer and die from so many health problems that could have possibly been avoided. So, this is why I have written this book. I know there are so many other *health and wellness* type materials on the market, but as we all band together in an effort to educate the masses, I am convinced that we can help many people. I do not claim to be a know-it-all, nor do I have all the answers, but I do know some things that have helped me and others. I would not be content or comfortable if I were to keep what I have learned all bottled up inside of me when there may very well be someone out there who may benefit from my knowledge and experiences related to health and wellness. It is my desire that several lives will be touched by the contents of this book. But, if only one life can be helped, if only one life can be saved, if only one life can be turned around, it would be well worth the time and effort that I have put into writing this material.

This book is not intended to condemn you or to make anyone feel guilty about their life. Instead, it is my hope that it would be viewed as a tool to use to help you, or someone you know, to incorporate a more healthier lifestyle, and to make and take the necessary changes to do so. It is also my desire that this book will be an inspiration to others as I share my personal and learning experiences as I travel on this ongoing journey of a healthy way of life. I want others to be encouraged in knowing that no matter their age or how unhealthy they may consider themselves, there is hope. Furthermore, to the best of my ability, I would like to show you, through the contents of this book, how achieving a healthy lifestyle can be accomplished. Please don't give up by not making and taking those steps towards living a much healthier lifestyle, because you can do it!

Beloved, I wish above all things that thou mayest prosper and be in health, even as thy soul prospereth.

3 John 1:2

Chapter 1

How My Journey Began

There are really two main events that happened in my life that placed me on this path of living a healthy lifestyle, and having such a sincere passion for others to do the same.

The first event happened in 1995 and it came as a total shock to me. It was the beginning of the last week in May. As I was about to get out of bed, before I put my left foot on the floor, the Lord spoke these words to me: "If you don't start exercising, you are going to die." I was startled, yet I knew why He said what He said. You see, I had been diagnosed with high cholesterol a few years prior. Never before had I engaged in a regular workout routine. But on this day, after hearing the Lord's words, I found some clothes I could work out in, put on my tennis shoes, and immediately went outside and walked around the backyard. I took a timer with me and set it for 20 minutes. The next day I did exactly the same thing; I walked around the backyard for 20 minutes. The third day, I attempted to do the same walk, but I had become bored already. With that, I broke out of the gate and began to walk in my neighborhood. I was living in Birmingham, Alabama at the time, and the area in which I lived had plenty of hills. I walked up and down those hills faithfully seven days a week. My walk totaled anywhere from three to four miles a day. It did not matter if it was cold, hot, raining or snowing, I was out there every morning. Since I had a daytime work schedule, I would start my walk around 4:00 AM each day. Many days, I would walk by myself. Other days, my husband, Phil, and/or one of my girlfriends, would walk with me. It became such a regular routine that the neighbors who were headed to work that early in the morning would honk their horns and wave as they passed me by. I carried with me a fanny pack fastened around my waist. In that fanny pack I had my cell phone, a note pad, an ink pen, gloves, a face towel and a hooded, paper-thin raincoat. I also carried a bottle of water.

I remember one morning it was raining so hard, but I continued to walk. I reached into my fanny pack, put on my raincoat and just kept on walking. When I got to the corner gas station where I would usually turn around and head back towards home, one of my neighbors who would pass me by every morning, was at the gas station pumping gas. He yelled to me, "One thing I will say about you is, you sure are consistent. Rain or shine you are out here." That really encouraged me because he spoke one key word and that was "consistent." I knew in order for me to accomplish what I was hoping to achieve, to lower my cholesterol, I had to be consistent.

I continued this walking routine for three years in a row – seven days a week. Even when we would go on vacations, I would find some way to include my walking exercise. After three years of what I thought would lower my cholesterol, I still received abnormal readings from the cholesterol tests. My reports continued to read that my cholesterol was high and that I should see a dietitian. I had seen a dietitian once and did not see any need to keep going back for her to tell me the same things she had told me previously. Needless to say, I was frustrated and felt that my diligence was all in vain, for my cholesterol continued to be high.

I could have easily gone on medication, but I did not want to. Matter of fact, I was talking to one of my friends about my frustrations with high cholesterol, and she suggested that I go see her "really good" doctor. I took her up on that and went to see her doctor. I had kept a record of all of my cholesterol test results for at least five years. When I showed them to him, he suggested putting me on a cholesterol lowering medication. I explained to him that I did not want to go on any medications, but instead I wanted to do what I could through "diet" and exercise. He alluded to the fact that obviously what I was doing was not working and this "low" dosage of the medication was not going to hurt me. I told him I did not want to become dependent on this or any other medication. Furthermore, I said, "Since this medication has side effects, chances are I would end up taking additional medication(s) for the side effects." He, of course, disagreed with what I said. This doctor and I went back and forth with this conversation, with him suggesting I try the medication and with me saying I did not want to try it.

When I left the examination room and went to the receptionist to check out, the receptionist handed me a bag of pills. It reminded me of a bag of *goodies* that I used to get when I went out trick-or-treating as a kid. As the receptionist handed me this bag of drugs, I told her that I had explained to the doctor that I did not want to take any medication. She told me the doctor wanted me to try them for just 30 days and then come back to see him. Realizing she was just the messenger, I accepted the bag of pills, but I never did take them. Also, I never did go back to see this particular doctor. (Note: I am in no way encouraging or suggesting that anyone should not take their medication(s), but what I am saying is that this is the choice that I made for myself).

After continuing to receive high cholesterol readings, I thought maybe I needed to start running. I have very flat feet, and as a result running takes its toll on my weak ankles. However, I was willing to do what I thought I needed to do in order to get my cholesterol down.

One day I was talking with my son, Paul, who was about 19 years old at the time. I was telling him how frustrating it had become, trying so hard to lower my cholesterol but yet continuing to get these high cholesterol readings. I told him I was going to start running outdoors. He suggested that I join the "Y" instead. It was a safer environment and there was more equipment there that I could use. I did just that. I became a member of the YMCA that was close to home. I would go to the "Y," work out, shower and get dressed from there, and head to work.

Approximately two years later, I was still getting high cholesterol readings. By this time I was really frustrated. I had been working out for about five years now and I was still getting the same negative reports. Once again, I was having a discussion with Paul, expressing my frustrations. He asked, "Ma, have you ever prayed about it?" It was like a light went off in my head. With some sense of embarrassment, I had to respond, "No." Here it was, about five years after the Lord had spoken to me about exercising, and I had not once confided in Him. I had not confided in Him about my frustrations or what He would suggest that I do because, so far, what I was doing on my own was not working. It was not that I was not praying for other things, but I just had not prayed about this particular matter.

It was during the mid to latter part of 2000 that I prayed to the Lord about *my* battle with high cholesterol. In January 2001, on a Saturday morning, as I was channel surfing on the television, I came across a Billy Blanks TaeBo® infomercial. I looked at the infomercial and thought, "I cannot do that." Then I said, "They are human. If they can do it, I can do it!" I then remembered that Phil and I had purchased a Taebo® videotape about a year prior that had never been used. So I went downstairs, popped the videotape into the VCR, and started doing Taebo®.

From the nutritional side, after discontinuing eating fried foods and many unhealthy foods, I later learned that dairy products, sugar, scallops, and shellfish in general (shrimp, crab and lobster) were causing my cholesterol level to stay elevated. So, I reduced my intake of dairy products, sugar, and eliminated all shellfish. In just four months after incorporating Taebo® into my workout routine and changing my eating habits when it came to fried foods, junk foods, dairy products, sugar and shellfish, I finally received a cholesterol reading of *normal*. It was a period of about eight years or more, from the time I first learned that my cholesterol level was high, to the time that I received a normal test result. I realize now just how much time I wasted by not seeking God's help in the first place.

Now for the second event that was instrumental in putting me on this health and wellness journey.

Somewhere around the period of time when I was dealing with high cholesterol, I was watching a television judge show one day. On this particular show, there was a sixteen-year-old boy who applied for a credit card by filling out an application that came in the mail, addressed to his father. After the boy received the credit card in the mail, he commenced using it. He purchased cell phones, pagers and other items for his so-called "friends." The father had no idea his son had applied for this credit card, so obviously he was unaware of him using it – at least until he received a bill for over $1,000. Since the father was responsible for paying the bill, he took his sixteen-year-old son to court for reimbursement of the payment he made on the credit card. In the courtroom was also this teenager's adult cousin. The cousin testified that she believed her young cousin made these purchases in an attempt to win friends. You see, the sixteen-year-old boy was extremely overweight.

It did not take long for this sharp judge to put two and two together. She took the sixteen-year-old into her chambers, without his father or his cousin. She asked him if he was picked on at school because of his weight — he replied, "Yes." She went on to ask him if he wanted to do something about his weight —

he replied, "Yes." As the tears rolled and the hurt was displayed on the face of this child, the judge told him about a camp for overweight teens that she could send him to, if he wanted to go. The boy said he was interested in going. In the meantime, the judge told him she was not letting him off the hook in regards to the money he charged on the credit card, where he used his father's name. She said if he had to rake leaves, shovel snow, or whatever, he was going to earn enough money to pay his father back.

I sat there and also wept as I saw the pain and the burden that this boy was carrying, all because of his weight. I wanted to reach out to this kid, put my arms around him and tell him, "I would like to help you, and I will." Of course, I could not do that, but that was where my heart was. Furthermore, I really didn't know back then what to do to help him, even if I could.

As time went on, the memories of what I saw in this child on that day did not go away. I felt a sense of helplessness that did not cease. Subsequently, a burning desire to help others with their health challenges began to increase, and that sincere desire would not and did not stop. I began to realize that if a healthy lifestyle is introduced during the early stages of a person's life, then unhealthy habits will become less likely to carry over into one's adulthood. On the other hand, I also recognized the fact that it does not have to be too late to start living a healthy lifestyle, regardless of an individual's age.

With what I learned while dealing with my own challenges with high cholesterol, coupled with what I saw on that judge television show that day, the seed of my health and wellness quest was planted. And, as with most seeds, as long as they are nurtured they will grow. As my interest in health and nutrition developed more and more over the years, I nurtured this seed by learning as much as I could about some of my own health issues, as well as other health-related subjects in general.

So now you have it. What you see here is the growth and development of that seed that was planted in me several years ago. Through this book, you are seeing the result of that burning desire to share with others what I have learned, and to do all that I possibly can to help as many individuals live longer and healthier lives. You are experiencing the outpouring of my heart's

deep and sincere passion for good health and wellness to flow
into and penetrate the lives of all people.

Chapter 2

My Personal Health Challenges

There are basically three ways in which we can live a healthier lifestyle. The first is to include prayer, and the other two are through nutrition and exercise. As I mentioned earlier, I had some health challenges. I am so very thankful to say that I have been blessed to have overcome most and shown great improvement in others. I can attribute all three of these ways: prayer, nutrition, and exercising to the reason as to why I improved or overcame certain health issues. See, I prayed about my situations, but there were still things in the natural I had to do. In this instance it was eating healthy and exercising.

High Cholesterol

The very first real health issue that I ever had to deal with in my life was high cholesterol. I was about 39-40 years old at the time. In the previous chapter, I went into specifics about how *I* battled this condition. Thank God for my son, Paul, reminding me to pray about it, and I thank God for sending answers to my prayers. Even though walking was the means of exercise that I started doing to reduce my cholesterol, and even though it didn't help it initially, I did receive a bonus when I started my walking routine. I lost 20 pounds. I went from a 12 dress size to a size eight, and I can even wear some size sixes.

Fibroid Tumors

I was next told I had fibroid tumors. Even though my doctor explained these are bound to occur as a woman gets older, taking care of the body through nutrition and exercise may reduce the possibility of having any problems as a result of them. After years of having fibroid tumors, I have not had any problems associated with them, and one of my doctors told me they are shrinking.

Torn Cartilage

The third health issue was, after having an MRI, it was discovered that I had torn cartilage (meniscus) in my left knee. The doctor wanted to do surgery to repair it. Well, just like I am not one who quickly takes medication, neither am I one who is quick to be cut on, so I quickly turned down the surgery. The pain in my knee was excruciating. Oh, it was an awful pain, it would hurt so badly.

This was around a year or two after I had started walking. But guess what? I just kept on walking, even though I was in pain. This pain went on for at least two to three years, but I was determined not to have surgery and I never took any prescription drugs for the pain. At that time, I didn't know much, if anything, about taking supplements. All I know, and all I can remember, is that it was very painful.

Well, over sixteen years or so later, I still have not had surgery on my knee and I no longer have the pain. I really don't recall exactly when the pain went away, but it's gone. I used to, from time to time, have little mild reminders of it, but nothing of any great pain like it had been at one time. In fact, in March 2006, x-rays were done on both knees and I was told that the cartilage in both of my knees looked very good. Also, now that I am more knowledgeable about supplements, I take certain ones for my joints, just as a precaution. I will go into more details on this when I discuss supplements. (Note: I am in no way encouraging or suggesting that anyone should not have surgeries, but what I am saying is that this is the choice that I made for myself).

Cold Hands, Cold Feet and Cold Nose

There was a time when I had extremely cold hands and feet, and the tip of my nose was always cold. I would dislike it every time I would have to shake someone's hand, because without a doubt, I was going to hear, "Oh, your hands are so cold." Some years after I started exercising, here again I can't say exactly when, I noticed that my hands and feet were no longer extremely cold, and neither was the tip of my nose.

Osteopenia

After having a bone density test in February 2006, I was diagnosed with Osteopenia. My doctor wanted to place me on a bone rebuilding medication. I went to another doctor and he suggested another type of medication to rebuild my bones. Well, I think you may know by now, I didn't take either one of the prescribed drugs. Now, here is a mistake I did make. By now I knew the importance of taking supplements, and I knew which supplements I should have been taking, but I didn't take them. I should have gotten on a good calcium supplement with vitamin D and magnesium. Well, in February 2008, I had another bone density test and the doctor (this was a different doctor in a different state), after looking at my 2006 test, said my bones had gotten worse. This doctor said (her opening statement was the same as all my doctors who get to know me), "I know you don't like to take medication, but..." She wanted to put me on an even different medication from the previous two. She gave a really good convincing speech as to why I should take it, so I told her to go ahead and call in the prescription. I even surprised myself this time. I actually told a doctor to phone in a prescription for me.

Well, after I got off the telephone with my doctor, I decided to do an Internet search on this medication. And, since I had previously been prescribed two other drugs used for Osteopenia, as well as for Osteoporosis, I decided to include them in my Internet search as well. After conducting the Internet search on these drugs, and as you become familiar with my track record on taking medications, do you think I ever picked up that prescription for bone rebuilding medication? You got it! Absolutely NOT! Those pills could still be sitting at the pharmacy, waiting on my arrival if they wanted to. All I know is that they were not going inside of my body! (Note: I am in no way encouraging or suggesting that anyone should not take their medication(s), but what I am saying is that this is the choice that I made for myself).

What I did do, however, is what I should have done back in 2006, when I was first told about my bones degenerating. I did pray about it back then, but I did not do what I should have done in the natural. That is, take the necessary supplements and include more strength training in my workout. Well, I started full force on the supplements and strength training in February 2008. Again, I will discuss more on the supplements as well as the strength training in the upcoming chapters.

In May 2009, I had another bone density test. This time by a third doctor, because I had moved to another state once again. The results of this exam showed my bones had not changed since my last bone density test. This doctor even told me there was not much difference between the three tests. He said my bones had not gotten better, but the good news was, they had not gotten worse. He also said he did not see any need to place me on medication. I have since had another doctor to tell me the same thing. Of course I was elated to get such reports and was glad I had never started on those medications that the previous doctors said I needed. I will just continue doing my strength training and taking my supplements, and I do believe whenever (or if ever) I have another bone density test, my bones will be in good shape.

It's interesting to note, even if I had taken the various medications for Osteopenia, my doctors were still recommending that I include calcium and vitamin D supplements on a daily basis. It seems to me that a person diagnosed with Osteopenia and Osteoporosis could possibly get the same results by taking supplements (in addition to eating right and exercising) without the use of medications.

Hot Flashes

In 2006, I started experiencing hot flashes. When I discussed the hot flashes with my doctor, he told me the best thing for them was to drink plenty of water and exercise. I told him that I do drink a lot of water and I exercise five days a week. He asked me, were the hot flashes mild or severe? I told him, when I have them, they are rather mild. He said if I was not exercising, they would probably be worse.

Fatigue & Insomnia

For a number of years, I had a problem with being fatigued and having symptoms of insomnia. I would get tired during the early part of the day, and at night I would fall asleep but have trouble staying asleep. I believe with prayer, the use of certain supplements, and making my nighttime atmosphere more conducive for sleeping, my sleep problems are constantly improving.

So here are just some of my health issues that were corrected, improved, or done away with altogether. I truly believe it is all as a result of: (1) Prayer, (2) Exercising and (3) Proper Nutrition (which includes supplements).

Chapter 3

Could You Be Playing Russian Roulette With Your Body?

The very first time I heard about and learned of the *game* Russian roulette was while attending college back in the early 1970s. This game was so named because it is said to have originated out of Russia, and it is patterned after the spinning of the wheel as in the game of roulette. Although I never actually played or witnessed the game of Russian roulette, I was surprised at what I learned as to how this game was played. I learned that this was a game where people would take a revolver containing one bullet and place the gun against their heads, usually right on the temple. They would then pull the trigger. If the bullet was not in the chamber when they had their turn to pull the trigger, then nothing happened. The gun was then passed on to the next person in the room. Then the next person would take their turn. When it came to the person who pulled the trigger and the bullet was in the chamber at the time the gun was fired, then the bullet would go straight into that person's temple. What happened next? In most cases, it was death. Sometimes instant death and other times a slow death.

The game of Russian roulette is what I see so many of us unknowingly doing to our bodies. No, we may not be placing a revolver to our heads or pulling the trigger like in the game of Russian roulette. But too many of us abuse our body by placing the wrong foods or unhealthy substances in it, and by not taking better care of it. In the game of Russian roulette, it's just a matter of time before the bullet will go off. In the game of life, it's just a matter of time before poor eating habits and neglecting or abusing our body will take their toll on us. In the game of Russian roulette, the unfortunate person who receives the bullet into the head may face death instantly, or may face a slow death. In the game of life, poor eating habits and the neglecting or abusing of the body may also result in instant death or a slow death. More likely than not, it is just a matter of time that an unhealthy lifestyle will affect the body in one way or another.

Why am I calling life a game? Well, just like in the game of Russian roulette, we are playing a game of chance with our lives. When we continue to eat the wrong types of foods, don't take proper care of our bodies, and/or abuse or neglect them, we treat our lives like a game, a game of chance. As we continue to keep on taking chance after chance by eating poorly, taking in harmful substances and abusing or neglecting our bodies, one day the unhealthy lifestyle is going to explode, just like that bullet in the game of Russian roulette. Our lives are not a game, and should not be treated as such, but instead our lives are a gift. This gift of life that God loves and so graciously gave to each and every one of us is so precious to Him.

Chapter 4

Designed for Destruction

There are certain foods that God designed for our bodies. These foods provide good nutrition for us and keep our bodies healthy. For the most part, these foods consist of fruits, vegetables, grains, beans, raw nuts and seeds. When we put these foods into our bodies, they know exactly what to do and where to go to nurture the body. On the other hand, when unhealthy foods such as sugar, fried foods, white flour, processed foods and all types of other "junk foods" enter into our bodies, they don't know where to go or what to do, so they just go all over the body, causing all sorts of problems. Why? It's because these foods were not designed for our bodies. Our bodies were not designed to reap any nutritional benefits from these types of foods because they were not designed by God for our eating.

I personally think that Satan saw "junk food" as a way, more so than any other way, that he could destroy our temples – our bodies. He designed these foods for our destruction...for the destruction of our bodies. Think about it this way. There are many things that so many people would not do because it goes against their moral principles and/or they view it as sin in the eyes of God. Such things as: fornication, committing adultery, telling lies, stealing, cheating, taking illegal drugs, drinking alcohol, or murder. These are some things that many people take a firm stand on and would not commit these "sins" for anything in the world. Yet, for some individuals, when it comes to food and taking proper care of the body, it's a totally different story a totally different stance is taken.

I believe Satan is having a good time, sitting back laughing at us as we destroy our bodies by not placing the proper foods into it and by not taking overall better care of it. From another viewpoint, I believe it grieves the Lord to see us purposely allowing certain things to destroy our bodies; things that He did not design for us to eat or do to our bodies.

There are certain foods that God placed on this earth for good nutrition. Let's take an apple, for an example. An apple in its natural form is very good for our bodies. It provides certain vitamins and minerals. It can aid in digestion, help with your joints, rid the body of toxins, etc. But when that same apple becomes a part of an apple pie, loaded with sugar and a pie crust made from white flour, the nutrients in that apple are destroyed. The apple no longer has the healthy value that it once had in its natural state – the way God created it.

Let's look at it from another perspective. The weather outside is all pretty with the sun shining. The sky is a beautiful blue and it's not cloudy at all. The birds are singing, the wind is calm and the temperature is just right. It's such a gorgeous day, so you decide to open up all your windows and all your doors to the house and enjoy the fresh outdoors. Because the winds are calm and it's a beautiful day, nothing on the inside of your house is going to be harmed or affected by you having all the windows and doors opened. The inside of your house is reaping all the benefits of the fresh outdoors.

Now, let's look at it like this. You have all of your doors and windows opened, but instead of a gorgeous beautiful day, it is a windy, rainy and a very severe stormy day. The winds are at 60 mph. Since all of the doors and windows to your house are opened, all of the effects from the outside winds and rain are coming into your house. These elements are causing havoc all throughout your house. Why? Because you gave them room to do so; you gave them an open invitation to come in and disrupt your house by leaving the windows and doors open under such severe weather conditions. You did not provide your house with the necessary protection by closing all of the windows and doors. Well, this is what we oftentimes do to our bodies. We allow the unhealthy elements to enter, and they cause all sorts of havoc throughout our temples – our houses – our bodies. We open the doors and the windows (our minds and our mouths) to our temples for them to be attacked by severe unhealthy conditions, by not providing them with the necessary protection needed. The necessary protection basically amounts to us taking proper care of our physical bodies through a combination of healthy eating and physical activity.

Chapter 5

Your Body is Very Valuable!

Certainly, there are environmental conditions we are faced with every day, but in most cases you and only you can determine what you put into your body and what you do to it. No one else has your body. Your body was assigned to you, but it belongs to God. Your body is the one and only one that God has given to you to live in while you are on this earth. God has not given anyone else the responsibility to reside in it but you and, of course, He desires to reside in it as well. Unless you are completely incapable of doing so, as an adult or young adult, no one else can physically take care of your body except you. In order for you to remain on this earth, you have to have a body to live in. A great deal of the condition of your body's residence depends upon you, and it's your responsibility to take control of its health. How you treat your body, what you do to it or what you do not do to it, is greatly affected by your choices. You are indeed your body's keeper! You are the one who has to look out for the best interest and the upkeep of it.

Suppose you were given a $200,000 car as a gift. The only stipulation — you must always put premium gas in the tank as suggested by the manufacturer. "Is that all?" you asked. "Yes," the gift-giver responded. You said, "Sure, that would be no problem whatsoever." The car was then given to you. Every time you gassed it up, you were very deliberate to put premium gas into the gas tank. You even took it a few steps further. On a regular basis, you made sure the car was kept clean on the inside and out. You got frequent oil changes and put nothing but the best oil in it. You treated it with tender loving care. One day you decided to put a lower grade of gas in your car. You quickly discovered that the car does not run as well with the lower grade of gasoline. After that one time of using the lower grade of gas, you vowed to stick to your word and only put premium gasoline in the tank from then on.

As mentioned in a previous chapter, our bodies are gifts from God. Just like the described gift car runs better on premium gas (as suggested by the manufacturer), our bodies operate better on those foods designed by our Manufacturer. Our bodies are a lot more valuable than that $200,000 vehicle. So much so that we can't even put a price tag on them. Our bodies deserve much more tender loving care than that vehicle, and a lot more of the deliberate attentiveness than the car. Even more so than the premium fuel we choose to put into the car's gas tank, our bodies deserve that fuel (food) that allows them to operate at their best. Yet, in some cases, more attention, care and concern would be placed on that car than on the body.

We can best take care of ourselves and our loved ones when we are in good health. We can best serve God and do what it is He has called us to do, when we are in good health. Our bodies are of great value to God, and therefore should be of great value to us. As a result, we should want to treat our bodies as such – very valuable! The individual body that each of us were personally given is ours and only ours for the duration of our lives. Do we nurture it with a healthy lifestyle, or do we abuse it with an unhealthy lifestyle? It is totally up to us how we choose to treat it, how we choose to nurture it, and how we choose to care for it. It's our own individual choice and our own individual call!

Chapter 6

The Natural and the Supernatural

Many times we are waiting on God to do things for us. Sometimes when things are not happening like we want them to, or within the time frame we desire, we want to blame God. But whatever we ask of God, there are some things we have to do as our part in the natural. For instance, let's say we have prayed and asked God for a job. We have faith in God and believe that God is going to provide the desired job. After all, we know God as being Jehovah Jireh, the One who provides! So with that, we sit patiently waiting every day for the phone to ring or for that special email to come through saying, "We have a job waiting just for you." Yet, in the natural, we are doing absolutely nothing to make any moves towards gaining employment. We have not submitted any applications, have not developed a resume, have not made any telephone calls, and have not even searched the Internet to see what jobs are available. "I'm just waiting on the Lord," is the only method used. We prayed to God for a job, in the name of Jesus, but in the natural, absolutely nothing was done and no action was taken on our part.

In Scripture, Jesus teaches us that we have a role to play in receiving from God. It takes us doing something on our part (the natural) in order for God to do something on His part (the supernatural). The natural and the supernatural have got to work together for us to see and to get results from God. John 14:13-14 states, "... *And whatsoever ye shall ask in my name, that will I do, that the Father may be glorified in the Son. If ye shall ask any thing in my name, I will do it.*" We must first ask, then God will do. We have got to first take action on our part (the natural) for God to then take action on His part (the supernatural).

How does this apply to our health? Well, some may be saying, "I have faith that God is going to heal my body." Or, "I have faith that no sickness or disease is going to attack my body." Yet in the natural, these people are smokers, and/or they eat nothing but unhealthy foods, they are "junk food junkies," they consume all drinks loaded with tons of sugar, and never drink any water. They open up their body to be attacked by the unhealthy elements, as discussed earlier. What are these people doing on their part so that their body can receive healing or so that sickness or disease cannot attack it? They are doing absolutely nothing! What are they giving God to work with? There is no way around it — we must take the necessary measures in the natural in order for God to take the necessary measures in the supernatural.

I would like to point this out. In the earlier scenario, I said some may be saying, "Well, I have faith that God is *going* to heal my body." The truth of the matter is, I believe we are not **going** to be healed, we are already healed. So oftentimes, people say they are praying for their healing, but we don't have to pray for healing because it has already been done. We don't have to pray for or ask God for something that is already ours; something He has already given to us. When Jesus went to the cross, He took on every sickness and disease. Isaiah 53:5 says, *"But he was wounded for our transgressions, he was bruised for our iniquities: the chastisement of our peace was upon him; and with his stripes we are healed."* 1 Peter 2:24, says, *"Who his own self bare our sins in his own body on the tree, that we, being dead to sins, should live unto righteousness: by whose stripes ye were healed."* In both of these books, Isaiah and 1 Peter, it clearly shows us that our healing is in the past tense. It was at the cross where our healing took place — because of Jesus

Christ, we are already healed. In the natural, we have to believe the Word of God, exercise our faith and receive our healing; not ask God for something He has already done for us. This is not to say one cannot get sick, but that through that sickness or disease, people should hold fast to their faith and stand firm on what the Word of God says, regardless of how the circumstances look or how one feels physically. Furthermore, while standing on the Word of God, continue to praise and thank Him for Who He is, for what He has already done, and for those things that are yet to come into your life.

It is my belief that it is not God's desire to see anyone sick. All throughout the Bible, we can see where Jesus' ministry included healing people, not making them sick. Acts 10:38 says it like this: *"...How God anointed Jesus of Nazareth with the Holy Ghost and with power: who went about doing good, and healing all that were oppressed of the devil; for God was with him."* This Scripture tells us that Jesus healed **all**, not some, but all. It also helps us to understand that sickness is of the devil and not of God. Hebrews 13:8 says that *"Jesus Christ is the same yesterday, today, and forever."* You see, the Lord has not changed. It is the same today as it was yesterday, that God's desire is for people to be healed and not sick or oppressed — Jesus bore all of that for us.

Throughout the first chapter of Genesis, we can see how God formed the entire world by speaking it into existence. In Genesis 1:26-27, it states, *"And God said, Let us make man in our image, after our likeness...So God created man in his own image..."* So not only did God create the world by speaking His words, but He also created us in His image. With that said, we can create our world and our conditions by speaking them into existence just like God did. Why? Because He said we were created in His image. If we continue to say we are sick, we will get what we speak, sickness. But when we speak the Word of God, such as, "By His stripes I was/I am healed," then we will receive just what we speak ...healing!

Yes, Jesus bore our sicknesses and diseases, and by His stripes we were/are healed, but there are still moves and responsibilities we have to make on our part. In the Bible, many times when Jesus healed, He told the recipients that it was their faith that made them well. Even though Jesus had the power to heal, the faith of these individuals was the connecting force to their healing.

Through their faith, they actually believed the healing they were seeking was a done deal. (Matthew 8:5-10; Matthew 9:27-30; Mark 5:25-34; Mark 5:35-42; Luke 6:17-19). Jesus still has the power to heal today but, in the natural, we have to exercise our faith and believe that we have already received our healing. We should believe and have faith in what the Word of God says we are, in this instance healed, and not what our circumstances look like or how we feel.

I stood on God's Word and believed and received, by faith, by the stripes of Jesus I was already healed of the various health challenges that I faced. But I still knew I needed to reach out to God to find out from Him what I needed to do in the natural to do my part. God's part was done when Jesus went to the cross, but my part had to be made known to me, so I sought God for His wise counsel.

Let's look back at the example about our job search. What do you think our chances would be of getting a job just by "waiting on the Lord," and not doing anything in the natural to gain employment? Now, what are our chances of living a healthier life just by waiting on the Lord and, in the natural, living an unhealthy lifestyle? In Matthew 7:7-8, Jesus said, *Ask,* (our part) *and it shall be given you;* (God's part), *seek, and ye shall find; knock,* (our part), *and it shall be opened unto you:* (God's part), *For every one that asketh receiveth; and he that seeketh findeth; and to him that knocketh* (our part) *it shall be opened* (God's part).

Again, we have responsibilities to fulfill in the natural. In the words of Pastor Kenneth Hagin, Jr., Senior Pastor of RHEMA Bible Church, "The natural and the supernatural coming together produce an explosive force for God!" When the natural and the supernatural come together, we get powerful results!

Chapter 7

You Can Eat Your Way to Good Health

Let's go down this imaginary journey. Suppose you have just come home from work. After a long day, you are very exhausted. Your desire is to lay your head down and rest for the remainder of the night. But before doing so, you want to take a hot bath and wash your hair. You fill the bathtub up with some hot water and you lay out the shampoo you are going to use to wash your hair, along with the oil you will apply to your body after you bathe. Before getting into the tub, however, you brush your teeth. You squeeze the paste onto your toothbrush and it is just that — all-purpose white paste. Now that you have completed brushing your teeth, you rinse your mouth out with some liquid pine-scented cleaner. You are now ready to get into your tub of hot water as you add 10 gallons of bleach to your bath water. You soak in the tub of hot water with the added bleach and then scrub your body down with the cleanser you added to your steel wool pad. Now it's time to shampoo your hair, but instead of hair shampoo you use carpet shampoo. Now that you have completed your bath, and the washing of your hair, you are now drying your body off with the towels that you recently used to wash your car. The oil you set aside, which is motor oil, is now applied to your body.

The truth of the matter is, we would not brush our teeth with an all-purpose white paste. We would not rinse our mouths out with a scented pine cleaner. We are not likely to add 10 gallons of liquid bleach to our bath water. We would not scrub our bodies with a steel wool pad with added cleanser. We would not shampoo our hair with carpet shampoo. We would not dry our bodies off with the towels we used to wash our car. And we would not rub our bodies down with motor oil. Why? Because we know these things are not good for our bodies. We know these products were not created or intended to be used on our bodies in this fashion. We are very careful and particular about what we put on the outside of our bodies and how we take care of and pamper them, so we would not use such harsh chemicals on any of the external parts of our bodies. Such chemicals used on the body's exterior would be pure self-inflicted abuse and cruelty.

Well, just as we are so careful, so attentive, so deliberate, and so particular as to how we care for the outside of our bodies, we should take that same care and concern for our insides. Some of the foods we eat may cause just as much damage, if not more, to the inside of our bodies as the chemicals described in this bizarre and ridiculous illustration. We would consider it bizarre and ridiculous to treat our external bodies with these products, but would we consider it to be bizarre and ridiculous if we were to inject them into our bodies by way of our mouths?

Suppose we could take those same chemicals described above, and smear them all over the insides of our bodies; all over the brain, the heart, and every other vital organ; all over every muscle, every tissue, every cell, every vein, every bone, every joint, and throughout the bloodstream. Well, because of what they contain, in essence that is what we are doing when we eat many unhealthy foods. Some foods are just as, or even more so, detrimental to the inside of the human body as these chemicals would be to the outer body. Eating unhealthy foods can cause damage and harm to our bodies, which may result in certain illnesses, sicknesses, diseases, health problems, and yes, even death. Just because the damaging results may not be as visible to the eye as they would be by using these harsh chemicals on the outside of our bodies, that does not mean the damage from eating unhealthy foods is not taking place on the inside.

I am convinced that all foods fall into two different categories — killer foods or healer foods. Obviously, the killer foods would be the unhealthy foods, and the healer foods would be the healthy ones. God created our bodies to be capable of healing themselves whenever the need arises. The body's healing process can best perform when it has been provided good nutritional, healthy foods, and afforded the opportunity to live in a healthy environment. Your body is your friend and your partner for life. It relies on you to provide it with what it needs to stay healthy, strong and self-healing.

I discovered that I am healthier when I eat fruits, vegetables, raw nuts, seeds and beans. When I started looking into these foods, I discovered that they contain a number of vitamins, minerals and other healthy nutrients needed to nurture the body. I had so often heard about antioxidants and free radicals and decided to find out exactly what they were and what they meant to my body. In a brief description, antioxidants are good for the body; they are a friend to the body. They help to keep the immune system — the body's built-in mechanism to protect it from the attack of illness — strong and healthy. Antioxidants also help to slow down the aging process and those illnesses oftentimes associated with aging. Free radicals, on the other hand, are an enemy to the body, they cause damage to the body, they break down and weaken the immune system, and they speed up the aging process and those health problems oftentimes associated with aging. I realize as we get older in years, we are faced with aging. But just because the number of our years increase as we advance in age does not mean we have to suffer, be stricken with sicknesses and diseases, or with any other sort of health problems. Aging does not have to have many of the unhealthy medical issues attached to it if we take good care of our bodies.

Glutathione

God placed an antioxidant substance into our bodies called glutathione. Some doctors, scientists and researchers refer to glutathione as the master or the mother of all antioxidants. Isn't that just like God to provide us with nothing but the best? Glutathione, the God-given, mother and master of all antioxidants, is a part of each of us. In addition to glutathione being the greatest antioxidant, it also helps to boost the immune system and rid the body of toxins. This substance called glutathione is adversely affected by certain conditions such as our environment, the unhealthy foods we eat, stress, **over**-exercising and aging. But there is hope. Increased levels of glutathione present in the body decrease the success of sicknesses and diseases attacking the body. A high level of glutathione enables the body to heal itself. We can boost our levels of glutathione in our bodies by eating healthy foods, doing regular exercise, but not over-exercising, because that can deplete the levels of glutathione, and taking supplements. Fish oil is one of the many supplements that help to increase the level of glutathione in the body.

My intentions herein, without going into a whole lot of details about glutathione, is just to make you aware (in case you are not already aware of it) of this great substance that is naturally produced in your body to help keep you healthy. I would highly recommend searching the Internet or going to the library to learn more about this master/mother of all antioxidants called glutathione.

More on Antioxidants

The antioxidants found in healthy foods such as fruits, vegetables, beans and some seeds and raw nuts, and even certain herbs and spices, also help to keep the body healthy and boost our levels of glutathione. As we place these antioxidant-containing foods into our bodies, we provide a safer, a healthier and — more likely than not — a longer life-containing vehicle for our bodies to reside. Antioxidants help to keep the cells in the body healthy, in good condition, and they help to fight off illnesses. Low levels of antioxidants give room for free radicals to reside and cause damage to the cells in the body, thereby increasing the chances for sicknesses and diseases to attack it. The human body has trillions of cells in it that make up every part of the body, including its vital organs (the brain, heart, lungs, etc.). Cells can very well be referred to as the building blocks of the body. Our cells are constantly dying and replenishing themselves, some even on a daily basis. It is my understanding that when cells die as good cells, they are going to replenish as good cells, but if they die as damaged cells, then they will replenish as damaged cells. The higher the levels of antioxidants placed into the body, the more antioxidants we have to produce and replenish good cells, to repair the damaged cells, and to fight off and absorb free radicals.

Free Radicals

Let's talk a little about that enemy to the body, free radicals. Free radicals destroy the good cells in the body, they break down the immune system, and they promote all types of sicknesses, diseases, and health problems. A good illustration often used to describe what free radicals do to the cells of the body is that of an apple. Once an apple is peeled, if not eaten right away, it will quickly start to turn brown. This browning process is known as oxidation. The longer that apple sits, the browner and less appealing it becomes; that oxidation has now destroyed the apple. Well, this is what free radicals do to the human cells. They destroy the good cells through this process of oxidation, they break down the immune system, and they pave the way for the attack of sicknesses, diseases, illnesses and various health problems. They function as a means to bring about destruction to the body's cells, thereby damaging the vital organs and other parts of the body. Think about it. Shouldn't we all want a body that contains a huge amount of good and healthy cells, versus one that houses a large amount of damaged and unhealthy ones?

Just like we get our antioxidants through the healthy foods we eat, free radicals are produced as a result of the unhealthy foods we choose to eat. Such foods as white breads, white pastas, white sugar, white rice, white flour, processed meats, processed foods, fried foods, and all other foods known as *junk foods*. In addition, lack of exercising and not taking certain supplements may promote free radicals in the body as well.

Practicing and Applying Healthy Eating

As much and as often as possible, I try to apply this principle to my life – *If it has or serves no nutritional value, then it is not going into my body.* I am not going to say that I never eat a piece of pie or a piece of cake or some other type of junk food, because that would not be the truth. But the intake of these types of foods is rather infrequent for me. There was a time when, on a daily basis, I ate more junk food and unhealthy foods than I ate what was good and healthy for me. Why? Because I did not know at the time what these foods were doing to my body. I didn't know the advantages of eating healthy and the disadvantages of eating unhealthy foods. And the truth of the matter is that they tasted good! But remember how I mentioned earlier how I believe the devil purposely designed unhealthy foods to destroy our temples? Well, why wouldn't he make them taste good? If he didn't, we might not eat them and he would not be able to tempt us or destroy our life-carrying vehicles with food. Anyway, I now limit that piece of cake to such special occasions like my birthday or anniversary – events that only happen once a year – and even then I don't overdo it. Whereas before, there was a time when I sincerely felt like my daily meals were not complete without some type of unhealthy dessert.

Another thing I try to practice is not bringing unhealthy foods into my house. No matter how much I may possibly crave a piece of cake at 10:00 PM, if it's not in the house I can't eat it. And the chances are very slim that I would hop into my car, right then and there, and go to the store to purchase a cake. However, what is more important to point out is that the more I started eating healthy foods, the less I craved the unhealthy ones.

You may live in a household with others who have not joined you in your healthy eating plan. They continue to buy the cakes, the pies, the potato chips, cookies, ice cream, etc. I realize this can be a real challenge. So what do you do in this instance? You may first try explaining to the person(s) what you are trying to accomplish...a healthy eating lifestyle... and ask them if they would help you by joining in on your endeavor. If they do, it becomes a win-win situation for each of you. If that fails, when you go into the kitchen and you are tempted to eat that cake or ice cream that they brought into the house, grab a piece of fruit and eat that instead. Oftentimes that will satisfy that sweet craving. In place of ice cream, I like to blend a ripened avocado in about eight ounces of (plain or vanilla) almond milk, a few pieces of frozen fruit, like cherries, a half banana, and a dash of cinnamon and ginger in a blender. Or, for a nice chocolate pudding, I mash an avocado and a half banana in a cereal bowl with a fork, and mix it with one heaping teaspoon of cocoa powder, about two teaspoons of almond milk, a half teaspoon of xylitol (a natural sweetener), and a few dashes of cinnamon and ginger. For the salt craving, try eating some veggies like carrots or celery. Spreading some cashew or almond butter (not the kind that contains added sugar) on a plain whole grain rice cake can help as well. At times, I like to even top it off with some raisins and chopped nuts. I also like to cut an apple into four pieces and spread some almond or cashew butter on each side of the individual slices. These are just a few of my favorite snacks, but when you use your creativity, you can create so many different healthy treats.

Not everyone can start eating healthy cold-turkey or instantly, and that's all right. Taking little steps one day at a time will get you on track. You may eat a dessert at each meal, like I once did. You can start by reducing that to a dessert once a day; then twice a week, then once a week then once every two weeks, until you have reduced it to perhaps those special occasions. This may seem a bit difficult at first, but the more you do it, the easier it becomes. After a while, whenever you may crave those sweets, you can reach for something healthy, like a piece of fruit instead of that candy bar. The good news is, after eating healthy for a period of time, not only does it become easier and easier to resist those foods that are not healthy for you, but you may find that you no longer have that strong desire for them like you once had. The key is to make and to take some steps (even little steps) on a daily basis until you have implemented and incorporated a healthy way of life for yourself.

It has often been said that a great percentage of many health problems come about as a result of a weak immune system. A weak immune system is oftentimes the result of poor eating habits. It has also been said that many health problems, including cancer, are a result of eating unhealthy foods, and have a greater chance of prevention through healthy eating. A weak immune system, caused by unhealthy eating habits, opens the door for a great number of health problems, while a strong immune system, as a result of healthy eating habits, shuts the door to many health problems.

Unfortunately, there are certain diseases that even healthy foods can do more harm than good. Just as one example, potassium is good for the heart and it helps to keep your muscles in good working order. It is the role of healthy kidneys to keep the right amount of potassium needed in the body. A person with an unhealthy kidney, or kidney disease, will often need to limit foods that can cause the level of potassium in their blood to increase to a dangerous level. Large amounts of potassium are found in such foods as: bananas, tomatoes, cooked broccoli, cooked spinach, etc. Potassium levels should be routinely monitored in order to determine if certain foods should be restricted. Your doctor can check the condition of your kidneys as well as your potassium level. If it is determined that the potassium level is too high, the kidney is unhealthy, or there is kidney disease, and certain foods should be limited or avoided, the body is robbed of some healthy foods that would have otherwise provided it with good nutritional benefits. If you do have a medical condition that can be adversely affected by certain foods, be sure to become familiar with those foods you need to limit or avoid. The good news is there are still many healthy foods that can be eaten to help nurture the kidney or any other part of the body that may have been affected by a health problem. Also, never give up on the belief that your body can be completely healed from whatever sickness, disease, or medical problem you may be dealing with.

The food industry has now bombarded us with so many unhealthy foods. Obviously, it's not because they are concerned with the health of people, but instead because it's a money-maker. Then, when people get sick, the drug industry can make money off the drugs that people buy, and take, trying to make themselves feel better and to get well. In both cases, the food industry and the drug industry are making money off the poor eating choices that many people choose to make.

Years ago, our food markets were small in size and consisted mainly of fresh fruits, fresh vegetables and fresh meats. Now the markets have become flooded with a wide variety of foods, mostly unhealthy, so that they are now known as "supermarkets." Over a period of time, our markets have become so huge that they had to increase in size to accommodate the housing of shelves and shelves of unhealthy foods. Just take a look around in your favorite "supermarket" and pay close attention to the types of foods it has made room to accommodate and made available for you to purchase. You will notice that our markets have grown in size as a result of several hundreds of unhealthy foods and drinks now being sold for our consumption. The number of unhealthy and bad food choices definitely outweighs the healthy and good food choices, and they can even be tempting and enticing to purchase. The best thing to do is to shop in the outer aisles of the store and not down the middle. The healthier foods are mostly found in the outer sections, or the perimeter of the store, and the unhealthy ones are down the center aisles. But here again, when grocery shopping, this becomes another opportunity to remind yourself – *If it has or serves no nutritional value, then it is not going into my body.*

Our Children Need Our Help
Through television commercials, store displays, and other means of advertising, the food industry is even attracting our children

with so many different unhealthy foods and drinks. As a result, we are seeing an increased number of overweight children. Additionally, the number of our children having poor medical conditions (and taking medications for those conditions) has increased in recent years. Many health problems such as high cholesterol, diabetes, high blood pressure, etc., used to be found mainly in adults, but is now being seen more and more in our children. The fact of the matter, however, is that parents and/or guardians can control what their children eat. The children are not the ones buying the food in the home, but it's the parents or some adult guardian.

As a parent or guardian, we should only want those foods to enter our children's bodies that are good for them, not those which can destroy them. We should insist on our children eating healthy, as well as incorporating some form of exercise into their lives. That way, when they become adults, those habits will be instilled in them and there's a greater possibility that they will adhere to what was embedded in them as children. Believe me, if this healthy lifestyle becomes a part of your children's lives while they are young, though they may not appreciate it during their youth, chances are when they become adults, they will love you for it.

I was reading the label of a so-called healthy food that kids can eat. The front of the package stated, "Enriched with Calcium, Build & Maintain Strong Bones, No Preservatives, No Artificial Sweeteners." On the front of the box of another product was stated, "7 Minerals and Vitamins." Wow! Both of these foods appeared to be something very healthy that we would want our children to eat, but that was not the case. When I read the actual ingredients of the first product, sugar was listed as its third ingredient and a form of monosodium glutamate (MSG), Hydrogenated Coconut Oil, was also listed. (Sugar and MSG are discussed in Chapter 8). In the second product, the one with the seven minerals and vitamins, it had a total of four ingredients listed. Out of those four ingredients, the second item listed was sugar and the third was high fructose corn syrup. These are only a few examples of the many processed foods and pre-packaged foods that have been disguised as healthy, but the truth of the matter is there is nothing healthy about them at all. Remember I mentioned earlier about the healer foods and the killer foods? Well, these are the kinds of foods that would fall under my killer foods category. What's so sad about it is that these are the types of foods that too many of our children are being fed on a regular and daily basis and under the pretense of being healthy foods.

Fast food restaurants have become a predominant place from which food is purchased for our children. Yet, many of the foods prepared at these restaurants are loaded with unhealthy fats, trans fatty acids, preservatives, MSG and sugar. Our children's bodies are being set up for destruction for the sake of what's been labeled as fast and convenient. The fast foods, the hot dogs, unhealthy pizza, macaroni and cheese, canned pastas, and the like, are doing more harm than good to our children. These types of foods are only preparing our children for an early death or a future of various health problems. It's so sad and so unfortunate, but the parents and/or guardians are allowing it. They are the ones buying into and supporting the demise of our innocent children.

I realize that oftentimes, processed foods are fed to our children because they are convenient, fast and easy to prepare. But once you get into the habit of preparing the **real** healthy foods, you will find they can be just as fast, easy and convenient. I think I can say, without a doubt, we all want our children to be healthy and well and not stricken with any of the various health problems that may develop as a result of eating poorly. It's not to say that a child should never ever have anything unhealthy, but it should only be on occasion, in moderation, not the normal way of eating but a rarity, and not fed as their main course or on a daily basis.

You may not have any children, or you may say you can't control what someone else feeds or want to feed their children, but this is how I have learned to handle that situation. There are some children whose parents feed them unhealthy foods the majority of time. If I am around them, and they want me to give or buy them some "junk food," I simply tell them, "I am not going to contribute to feeding you unhealthy foods. Instead, I will give/buy you something that's good for you." This may seem rather harsh to a child. But when I know most of the foods and drinks they consume are unhealthy, processed and pure old junk, I cannot, in good conscience, give them more unhealthy foods or drinks to ruin their delicate immune systems. It's also important to note that I would not call a child a negative name or say negative things about them that would perhaps attack their self-esteem. Instead, I try to give them encouraging words like, "I love you so much and care a lot about you. I want to see you grow up to be a healthy man/woman." I not only tell or teach them about being healthy, but I try to show them what it means to live healthy by being an example. As parents, guardians, relatives, or friends to our children, we are the only example they may have. We have to be the judge as to whether or not we are going to instill in them and teach them about having a healthy lifestyle. In addition, are we going to feed their precious bodies foods that serve as healing agents, or those foods that serve as killers? The choice is ours.

Another thing to note when it comes to our children is to watch for possible eating disorders. If you discover your child is eating certain foods and hiding the products' wrappers behind the curtains, under the furniture or cushions, don't ignore this behavior. On the other hand, you may have a child who does not want to eat, so they hide the actual food in these same places. In either case, this may be an indication of some type of food disorder, and it should not be overlooked. This is something that you should address with your child and not act as if it does not exist. Talk to your child, not in a scolding way, and try to find out why they feel they need to hide these wrappers or food. However, I would highly suggest speaking with a person who is a professional in dealing with eating disorders, to see what would be the best way to approach these types of behaviors. In doing so, it may very well prevent some long-term or future problems.

One good thing that is now required of the food industry is to list the ingredients on the labels of the foods they produce. It is so important to read the labels on the foods you buy and eat. In reading a food label, I pay particular attention to the calorie content, the type of fat, the amount of sodium and all of the ingredients listed. The government now requires the amount of trans fat to be included on food labels. Trans fat is a chemical process whereby liquid fats are made into solid fats through the hydrogenation (combining or treating an unsaturated substance with hydrogen) of oils. Trans fat is a harmful ingredient that is used to enhance the flavor of food and preserve its shelf life. Currently, trans fats/trans fatty acids are a hot topic of discussion as being something we need to avoid eating because of the various health problems they can cause. Even eating the smallest amount of trans fat can be very harmful to the body over a period of time. If you are ever in doubt about whether or not a food contains trans fat, if it's not in its natural state, if it is processed, and/or if it's cooked in unhealthy oils, chances are it contains trans fat. Also, as a rule of thumb, if the ingredients listed on a label are extremely long, with words that I don't understand or can't pronounce, then I know it is probably a food I would want to avoid. In addition, I try to avoid those foods that contain sugar, trans fat, MSG, high fructose corn syrup, and other added sugars and artificial sweeteners.

As I mentioned earlier, I mostly eat fruits, vegetables (a great amount raw), beans, raw nuts and seeds. I also eat brown rice, quinoa (pronounced keen-wah) and whole grains, which includes whole grain bread. My fruits and vegetables are either fresh or frozen. I mainly avoid buying canned fruits and vegetables because of the additives, excessive amounts of sodium, sugars and MSG that many of them contain.

One of my favorite breakfast meals is a healthy smoothie. My smoothie consists of about eight ounces of non-dairy milk like rice or almond milk, (water can be used in place of the milk), a combination of fresh and frozen fruits, (I like to mix and match some — not all at one meal — fresh apples, fresh oranges, fresh bananas, fresh grapes, fresh peaches, fresh or frozen: strawberries, blueberries, blackberries, cherries, cranberries or pineapples), about a teaspoon of cinnamon, a dash of ginger, a teaspoon of xylitol, three teaspoons of Bragg's Apple Cider Vinegar, a tablespoon of olive oil (extra virgin), and two tablespoons of flax seeds. At times, I may even add some fresh spinach and raw nuts.

With about six ice cubes, I blend all these ingredients in a blender. This smoothie is very filling and it provides me with a great amount of fruits I need and a portion of my vegetables when the spinach is added. When I purchase my frozen fruit, I always read the label to see if it includes anything else other than the fruit. For instance, the ingredient listed for the frozen strawberries is just strawberries and nothing else. There are some frozen fruits containing other ingredients as preservatives or sweeteners that I choose to avoid.

As another one of my favorite breakfast meals, I like to eat whole grain oatmeal. I specify whole grain, and not instant, because the instant has been processed, stripped of the grain's natural nutrients, and often contains some form of sugar. I cook my oatmeal on top of the stove with a non-dairy milk. After it is cooked, I mix in about two-three teaspoons of cocoa powder. I may also add some chopped nuts or blueberries. When purchasing cocoa powder, here is another instance where I read the label to make sure there is nothing else listed, because I want pure cocoa. The oatmeal is good for lowering cholesterol and the cocoa helps to keep the arteries clean and the blood pressure down. Even though I have never had a problem with my blood pressure, I still like to do those things to and for my body that will keep it in good working condition. Finally, I sweeten my oatmeal with xylitol or raw organic honey. Some days I may blend my oatmeal and cocoa powder in with my smoothie and take it all in at the same time.

Another good thing I like to make with pure cocoa powder, or dark unsweetened chocolate, is hot chocolate. I heat about a cup of rice, coconut, almond or hazelnut milk and mix in two-three teaspoons of cocoa powder or one square of pure dark unsweetened chocolate. I sweeten to taste with xylitol or raw organic honey, and then enjoy a good cup of hot chocolate.

I also like to juice fresh fruits and raw vegetables. One of my favorites is juicing carrots, apples and celery. This may not sound all that appetizing, but it is really a delicious and healthy drink. You can be creative and mix various raw veggies and fresh fruits together or separately. Since the juices contain the good nutrients from the fruits and vegetables, the liquid form that juicing provides enters into the bloodstream very quickly. Juicing fruits and vegetables can really provide many health benefits. I have heard of cases where individuals were dealing with some serious health issues and they turned to juicing and received miraculous results. For instance, I saw on a television health show where a lady had been diagnosed with stage four cancer. The doctor told her to go home and get her business in order with her family because she had less than a year to live. She said she prayed about it and the Lord led her to juicing. She started nurturing her body with the fresh fruits and vegetables she juiced. Needless to say, the lady was later tested and there were no signs of cancer.

The Friday night after Thanksgiving of 2009, we decided to have a juicing party at our home with family. My brother, Keith, made some coconut milk from two fresh coconuts. Then I juiced carrots, celery and apples. My next drink was the juicing of all fresh oranges. Finally, my brother topped it off with a berry mix drink which consisted of juiced: fresh strawberries, cranberries, blackberries, blueberries, oranges, kiwi fruit, apples, and in a blender, papaya. He mixed the papaya in with the fruit juices that had been juiced. Each of us had an opportunity to sample the coconut milk, then the carrot drink, then the orange juice and finally the berry juice blend. This activity was very timely after having such a typical big Thanksgiving meal the day before. Plus, it was something healthy that everyone could participate in and reap the health benefits as well. We really had a lot of fun doing this and everyone, including the kids, tasted the various drinks. I am seriously considering making a juicing party an annual event the Friday after Thanksgiving. It was a great time for family fun, food and fellowship!

Please note: There is a difference between the use of a blender and a juicer/juicing. The blender will blend up all the ingredients that you place into the blender, whereas a juicer extracts the juice and separates it from whatever fruit or vegetable you are juicing.

I am often asked what kind of seasonings I use in my foods. If I prepare some type of greens such as collards or kale, and dried beans like pinto beans, I like to cook them in about a tablespoon of extra virgin olive oil, and a variety of herbs and spices. To give them some extra flavor, I may add some green peppers, garlic, basil and/or onions. I like to sauté fresh spinach by adding a little extra virgin olive oil (just enough to coat the bottom of the skillet) to the pan and add some chopped garlic. At times, I will cook my spinach without adding olive oil or any other liquid, and allow it to cook in the water that it naturally contains. Fresh lemon or fresh lime juice and Bragg's Apple Cider Vinegar also make good seasonings.

I also like using organic extra virgin coconut oil to sauté foods in. This is what I use in place of vegetable oil or some type of shortening. In addition to its use for cooking, coconut oil can also be taken on a daily basis for its many health benefits. It is great for the skin too!

There are times when I like to purchase organic foods. Even though buying organic is my preference, I don't always buy organic because it can be rather expensive. However, whenever possible, I highly recommend that you purchase the healthy organic foods.

A few years ago when I started buying organic, I assumed that all organic food meant it was healthy food. I quickly learned that was not the case. Just because it is organic does not mean it is healthy. The same holds true for health food stores and foods that claim to be natural. Just because a store goes under the heading of "health food store" does not mean all the foods they carry are healthy, and a food saying it has natural ingredients does not necessarily mean it is healthy. There are many unhealthy organic foods on the market, there are many unhealthy products in "health food stores," and there are many "natural" unhealthy foods. That is why it is so important to read all food labels very carefully.

Something that works for me in helping to eat healthy is to keep my fruits visible. I have them sitting out in my kitchen, looking me straight in the face every day. If they are out of sight, like in the refrigerator, they can be out of mind. Anyway, if I crave something to snack on, I may quickly reach for an apple or some other kind of fruit. Speaking of apples, there was a time, during my mostly junk food eating days, when I did not like apples. I just did not like the way they tasted. When I made up my mind to eat healthy, I made myself acquire a taste for apples because I knew they were good for me. There may be some healthy foods that you just don't care for, but try telling yourself, "I'm going to make you eat this because I know it's good for you." It worked for me with the apples, and I'm so glad that it did.

When buying fresh fruits and vegetables, I try not to buy too much at a time because if not eaten fast enough, they will spoil, and that results in just pouring money down the drain. Furthermore, the longer certain fruits and veggies sit, they start to lose many of their nutrients and they won't provide all the health benefits they once had.

I try to cook just enough food for a particular meal, but there are times when I have leftovers. To store the leftover foods, I use glass jars or glass containers. When placed in the refrigerator, I try to keep them towards the front. This way they won't get lost or forgotten. Prior to implementing this process, I would put leftovers into the refrigerator in non-glass containers and forget all about them being there. Weeks later, I would discover the leftovers and they would be unfit to eat because they would have spoiled. With the glass container, the food stands out and I know it's something that should be eaten relatively soon. To reduce the accumulation of bacteria, it is best to eat leftovers within 48 hours of refrigerating. If they are not eaten within that time period and you want to save them for later, if they are a type of food that can be frozen, then they should be placed in the freezer. In addition to storing my leftovers in glass containers, I also cook in glass, stainless steel or cast iron cookware. Due to the harmful chemicals that can be released from the non-stick cookware, I choose not to use them.

I am constantly looking for and coming up with new and creative ways to eat healthy and to get into my body a sufficient amount of fruits and vegetables. Eating healthy foods is by far the best choice to make if you want to live a longer, much healthier life. As that saying goes, "You are what you eat." If you eat healthy foods, you will be healthy. If you eat unhealthy foods, you will be unhealthy. It is just that simple. It's just a matter of time before unhealthy eating habits will take their toll on the body, wear it down and induce some type of health problem(s) in an attempt to destroy you. On the other hand, healthy eating will do you and your body good!

Imagine if you could take a paintbrush, dip it into healthy or unhealthy foods, and paint all over the inside of your body with those foods. Well, in essence this is what we do when we place foods or other substances into our bodies. Whatever these foods or substances contain, whether good or bad, they are saturating all of the various parts and functions of our bodies.

Don't allow the food and drug industry to use you as one of their money-making machines by constantly consuming and making poor food choices which may, in turn, lead to you having to take some type of medication for relief.

Below is a list of some healthy foods to *"paint"* the inside of your body with. Keep in mind it does not include all healthy foods. Also, there are some foods that have a variety of healthy foods within their food group, for example there are many different kinds of apples.

- Apricots • Apples • Avocados • Bananas • Berries
- Blackberries • Blueberries • Cherries • Cranberries
- Grapefruits • Grapes • Lemons • Limes • Melons • Oranges
- Pears • Peaches • Pineapples • Plums • Raspberries
- Strawberries • Watermelons • Artichokes • Asparagus • Beans
- Beets • Broccoli • Cabbages • Carrots • Cauliflower • Celery
- Chives • Cucumbers • Eggplant • Garlic • Leafy Greens
- Lettuce (the darker green the better; Romaine instead of Iceberg lettuce) • Onions • Paprika • Parsnip • Parsley • Peas
- Pumpkins • Radishes • Raw Nuts and Seeds • Shallots
- Spinach • Sweet Potatoes • Tomatoes • Turnips

As you can see from the above list, we have a variety of healthy foods from which we can choose to eat. Use your creativity. Mix and match foods to come up with creative healthy snacks and meals.

The best way for me to define healthy foods (also known as whole or real foods) are those foods that are as close to their natural state in which God created them for our consumption. The unhealthy foods are those that have been altered from His original design and packed with all sorts of additives and preservatives and processed beyond their original state. So, if and when temptation arises, before consuming certain foods, I ask myself, *"What nutritional value does this food serve or have for my body?"* If the answer is "None," then, most of the time, I will choose not to consume it. Since I have practiced this habit for a while now, there are very few times when I have to ask myself this question. But there are occasions when I have to remind myself: *"If it has or serves no nutritional value then it is not going into my body."* I challenge you to adopt this principle. More often than not, you may be surprised at the decisions you make on the foods you choose to eat and/or those you choose not to eat.

I have heard so many people claim that because they have a family history of certain health problems, they are going to have them as well. This does not have to be the case. First of all, since we have the ability to speak things into existence, we want to be very careful not to speak any health problems into existence. Secondly, if we are aware of certain health problems running in our families, that should motivate us even more to want to take good care of our bodies. On the other hand, there are so many people who could have very well been born with strong healthy genes, but end up destroying them with the unhealthy choices they prefer to make.

If you do have any health problems, you can actually eat to improve your health. You can eat to reverse poor health conditions to good health by making healthy food choices and not the unhealthy ones. Make them, take them, apply them, claim them, saturate your body with them, and identify them as part of your healthy lifestyle for the rest of your life. Do this for a lifetime and not just for a particular event or for a particular moment, and chances are you will enjoy a better quality of life, a healthier life and spend more days feeling good and well as a result.

Chapter 8

The Dangers of Sugar & MSG

I am oftentimes questioned about ways in which a person can live a healthier lifestyle. One of my main responses, from the nutritional side, is to omit eating products containing sugar and MSG (Monosodium Glutamate). The most frequent response to the sugar is, "Well I don't eat a lot of sweets." In most cases, the response to MSG is, "What's that?" Please note, in this instance I am speaking of refined sugar products, and artificial sweeteners, and not the sugar that comes from eating fruits and vegetables. These healthy enriched foods, fruits and veggies, contain some form of natural sweeteners along with other vitamins and minerals that are good for the body. Some healthy natural sweeteners are: raw honey (preferably organic), stevia, agave nectar and xylitol. My favorite just happens to be xylitol. I like the way it tastes, plus it's easy on and good for the teeth. However, even with natural healthy sweeteners, they should be eaten in moderation because they do contain calories.

Although it is true that most unhealthy sweets contain some form of "bad" sugar, it is not just found in the obvious products, like candy, ice cream, pies, cakes, cookies, soft drinks, fruit drinks, etc., but it is also found in many of the not so obvious food products. Such foods as: cereals, breads, white rice, white flour products, white pastas, ketchup, barbecue sauce, mayonnaise, salad dressings, crackers, instant oatmeal, some so-called nutritional bars, many canned foods like soup, some spices, various types of chips, artificial sweeteners, processed meats (hot dogs, bologna, turkey, chicken, salami, bacon, sausage, etc.), chewing gum, and the list goes on. Here is another reason why it is so important to read food labels. Most processed foods contain some form of unhealthy sugar, trans fat, MSG, or a combination of all three. Even when we purchase ready prepared meats from the grocery store, like roasted chicken, chances are they contain a form of sugar(s) and/or MSG. The seasoned frozen meats that may taste so good to the taste buds are oftentimes loaded with sugar(s) and/or MSG. Some sugars and/or MSG are even contained in some baby foods, as well as formulas.

There are a number of names for unhealthy sugars. They may be listed on a food label as sugar, corn syrup, high fructose corn syrup or brown sugar, just to name a few. The MSG may in fact say Monosodium Glutamate, however there are other hidden names for it as well. Such names as hydrolyzed vegetable protein, hydrogenated coconut oil, autolyzed yeast, textured protein, etc.

About the only thing that foods containing sugar and MSG can do for the body is to satisfy that hunger feeling, while at the same time causing all sorts of havoc throughout the body. The feeling of hunger can easily be satisfied through those foods, here again, that are in their closest form in which God created them and placed on this earth for our consumption. Those foods containing a form of unhealthy sugar and/or MSG are creating more and more health problems. We should make every effort to avoid these types of foods as much as possible. The dangers of these two substances have become so pronounced that we are now seeing more and more food labels saying "sugar free" or "contains no MSG." (Note: Be careful of the "sugar free" products, because oftentimes they have been replaced with some form of artificial sweetener that is a form of MSG in disguise). Some restaurants are now even stating on their menus that their foods have no MSG. My husband and I recently visited a restaurant that had "We Hate MSG" printed on the front of the menu.

I could very well list several ways in which sugar and MSG cause danger to the body, but simply put, I would venture to say the consumption of sugar and/or MSG-containing products are the underlying cause of many health-related problems. I highly recommend anyone who may be facing some type of adverse health issue to eliminate sugar and MSG-containing products, and see if they don't notice and feel an improvement in their body. It could be a battle with cancer, inflammation, problems with the bones, joints, digestive problems, obesity, heart issues, any one of the organs, constant headaches, migraines, asthma, hyperactivity (particularly in children), certain allergies, etc., but the elimination of sugar and MSG could make a tremendous improvement and difference in one's overall health. Matter of fact, MSG and sugar are said to be like a fertilizer to cancer, as well as some other diseases. Cancer cells can lay dormant in the body. By eating unhealthy foods, those cancer cells can be activated. I don't think there is anyone who wants to have cancer of any sort, so why should we even want to create an environment for our bodies in which cancer and other health problems can flourish? Since cancer and other chronic diseases thrive on sugar and MSG, I would think the wise thing to do would be to starve these diseases. Since these chronic diseases don't like and don't survive in environments that are loaded with healthy foods like fruits and vegetables, starve them by loading the body with healthy nutrients. In addition, cancer and other chronic diseases do not like oxygen, and exercising helps to improve your body's intake of oxygen. Even if you are not facing any chronic health problems, it is so worth working towards eliminating sugar and MSG from the foods you eat, and of course to exercise. Healthy eating and exercising can help to reduce your chances of those unwanted, disease-containing, life-destroying creatures taking over your body.

Rather than going into great detail about the different types of dangerous sugars, as well as MSG, or the negative effect they both can have on the body, my intent is to bring these types of issues to your attention so that you can be aware of them, (in case you are not aware of them already), so that you can do your part to avoid their consumption, and to further look into and verify what I am saying through the use of the Internet and/or the public library's resources. I highly recommend doing some further research on the dangers of sugar and the dangers of MSG. Even if you don't want to believe what you find, give it a try by eliminating products containing these substances, and see if you don't notice improvement in your health. As you do your research, become familiar with the various names of "bad" sugars and MSG. That way you will be aware of them as you make your various food selections. I believe you will find the elimination of sugar and MSG-containing products, which include processed foods and trans fat, and eating the healthy-type foods discussed, will be well worth it. I am confident that your body will thank you!

Chapter 9

A Healthy Weight Loss Plan

Many of us have experienced being on an overcrowded bus, and it's not a pleasant feeling. Imagine, because of the crowdedness, you have to stand up on a bus and hold the overhead rail in order to keep from falling. As you are holding onto the rail, the person on each side of you continues to bump up against you. You are very uncomfortable as you are knocked to and fro. You feel like one of the many sardines in a can. You can hardly breathe, you can't move freely and you feel smothered. You know, without a doubt, you could function so much better if you were not under such confined and restricted conditions. You are longing for the time when you can get away from and be free of that undesirable environment. Well, this crowded, uncomfortable, and smothered feeling is an example of what our organs are experiencing when they are surrounded by excessive body fat. Just like we know we could function so much better if we were not on the bus under the conditions described above, the same goes for our organs.

They could function so much better if their surroundings were not invaded. Could it be, just like we would long to be free from that unpleasant environment on the bus, our organs are longing to be free from that environment that is smothering and crushing them as a result of excessive body fat? I would think so.

Obesity is becoming too much of a part of many lives today; not only in adults but in young adults and small children as well. I believe it would be safe to say that each of us has someone who is very dear and close to us, or who we love deeply, who is faced with excessive body weight. When one has a weight problem, it can be a rather sensitive subject for discussion. It is often a topic that is avoided because of this sensitivity. Although this sensitive subject is not easily approached, the truth of the matter is it's a real issue with serious and even life-threatening consequences. Obesity can lead to so many health problems. Just to name a few, there is diabetes, heart disease, liver and other vital organ problems, cancer, high blood pressure, joint problems, and yes, even an early death. When individuals are overweight, they put their entire life at risk. They may also be faced with many medical bills due to extra doctor visits, hospital stays and prescription medications that they might not otherwise need if they were not overweight. Even though I don't believe it's right, they may even be subjected to unfair treatment when it comes to employment opportunities, as well as having to pay higher rates for certain insurances.

As sensitive as the discussion of being overweight may be, if you were to see a car load of people about to drive down a dark road that led to a cliff with a 200-foot drop, would you warn them of that cliff at the end of the road, or would you just allow them to go down that road, knowing what they were about to encounter? Without a doubt, I would venture to say that most, if not all, of us would do what we could to warn them ahead of time. We would not want to see them or anyone else travel down that road to disaster.

What I am attempting to do in this chapter, as well as throughout this entire book, is to let people know there is help for many health issues they may be facing, even obesity. I know there are those who say it's all right to be overweight, and they are perfectly satisfied with the way they are. As with any situation, we have a right to choose what we believe or don't believe; what we want to do or what we do not want to do. We have a right to keep on doing what we have been doing and keep getting the same results, whether good or bad. Many weight problems are a result of lack of physical activity and food addictions that one may overcome by applying the principles outlined in this book. I hope that anyone faced with a weight problem will at least give what I am suggesting in this chapter, and throughout this book, a sincere try. If you don't want to do it for yourself, at least do it for those who love and care for you and want to continue to have you around in their lives.

One of the first keys to successful weight loss is to have a change of attitude and to renew the mind. You have to make up in your mind that this is what you are going to do. You have to gear your mind into a new way of thinking about your food choices and your physical fitness. Once you get your mind made up to lose weight, your body will come on board. If you are having difficulty with getting into the frame of mind that you are going to lose weight, and you are going to do the things to make it happen, then pray about it. Ask the Lord to help you with this desire you have, and to give you the strength to endure. Whatever you do, don't beat yourself up about your weight, or any medical condition you may have for that matter. Losing weight, maintaining a healthy weight, and doing those things to make that happen, may not be all that easy to do, but it can be done, especially if you pray about it and get your mind on board with the plan.

In essence, the way to achieve healthy weight loss is basically what has already been discussed in the previous chapters on healthy eating, exercising and, because they promote weight gain, avoiding foods containing MSG, trans fat, and processed sugars. However, below I have summarized a formula for losing weight in a healthy manner.

<u>Formula for Healthy Weight Loss</u>
1. Prayer. First pray and ask the Lord to renew your mind about food and exercising. Pray for the strength to resist those foods that are not healthy, and the desire to incorporate exercising into your life.
2. Eat healthy foods.
3. Cut down on food portions.
4. Track calorie intake.
5. Exercise.

6. Keep a journal of the foods you eat, the time of day eaten, and any exercise performed.

7. Discuss your meal plan and exercise program with your professional health care provider.

8. Be patient and don't give up!

Eat Healthy Foods

1. Fruits. Eat preferably fresh or frozen (not canned). Read the labels to make sure the frozen fruits only contain the fruit and not any additives. Bananas should be eaten in moderation during the weight loss plan. A half banana works for me.

2. Vegetables. Eat fresh or frozen vegetables (not canned). Read the labels to make sure the frozen vegetables contain only the vegetables and not any additives.

3. Brown rice

4. Grains such as: quinoa, oats, barley, rye, and whole wheat.

5. Whole wheat products like breads and cereals (be sure to read labels). When I eat bread, I limit it to one slice of wheat or whole grain a day. Some days I don't eat any bread at all.

6.   Sweet potatoes

7.   Juiced fresh fruits and vegetables.

8.   Blended fresh or frozen fruits and vegetables (like that of a smoothie).

9.   Fish, chicken or turkey (Prepare: baked, broiled, boiled and not fried. Avoid processed or pre-seasoned when purchased). It is best to eat organic meats to avoid the antibiotics and hormones found in most non-organic meats.

10. Eggs — Preferably organic and free range. (Not egg substitutes because of the additives so many of them contain).

11. Dried or frozen beans. (Be sure to read labels to avoid any additives to the frozen beans). Before cooking them, I like to soak the dried beans overnight. The next day I may add a mixture of fresh vegetables such as onions, celery, green peppers and garlic — to make a nice vegetable broth — along with a variety of herbs and spices. With just enough water to cover the ingredients, I would then place the beans, vegetables, herbs and spices, into the refrigerator for another night. The following day, I may add about a tablespoon

of extra virgin olive oil and cook slowly (on low heat) until the beans are tender. Even though this is an additional two-day process, it gives the vegetables, herbs and spices a chance to really get down into the beans and enhance their taste.

12. Drink half your body weight of water on a daily basis. Example: 150 pounds of body weight equals an intake of 75 ounces of water daily.

13. At least three cups of green tea a day. (To get the greatest benefits, do not add any type of sweetener to the tea — drink it unsweetened). One of the many benefits of green tea is that it helps to increase your body's metabolism. High metabolism increases the body's ability to burn calories. Green tea also contains antioxidants.

14. In moderation, natural sweeteners like stevia, xylitol, agave nectar or raw honey (preferably organic).

15. Raw nuts and seeds. Limit the serving size to about one ounce, or about 12 nuts, per serving. Soak them in water to remove the enzymes so that your body can digest them better.

Foods to Avoid

1.   White potatoes

2.   White rice

3.   White bread

4.   White pasta

5.   Any food made from or containing white flour

6.   Dairy (including cheese)

7.   Nuts or seeds cooked in oils, salted or sugar-coated

8.   Fried foods

9.   Fast foods

10. Any kind of *junk food*

11. Sugary foods and drinks, i.e., cakes, cookies, pies, candies, soft drinks, fruit drinks, ice cream, etc. Note: Eating white potatoes, white rice, white bread, white pasta, white flour, and white flour products is like eating unhealthy sugar.

12. Artificial sweeteners—many of these sweeteners are forms of MSG

13. Shellfish

14. Processed meats

15. Any food containing MSG

16. Foods containing trans fat

17.   Other processed and boxed foods, including crackers and other similar snacks.

Other Tips

1.   Have an accountability partner(s). This may or may not be someone who is also on the healthy weight loss plan, but it should be someone you would stay in constant contact with to report your progress and share your challenges. Make sure it is a person who has a positive attitude, is an encourager and is a true cheerleader for your success. You and your partner(s) would determine how often you communicate, but it should be frequent.

2.   Exercise a minimum of three times a week. Include strength/resistance training and cardio/aerobic exercise. Start slowly and gradually increase your intensity and duration.

3.   Reduce salt intake. (When eating salt, use sea salt). The amount of salt you eat, if you are trying to lose weight or not, should be limited to 2,300 milligrams (mgs.) per day. This is equivalent to about a teaspoon. Too much salt can cause high blood pressure, heart disease

and other health problems. Be sure to read food labels for salt (sodium) content.

4.   Try to complete your meals at least three hours before going to bed. You want to give your food a chance to digest and you want to have time to burn some calories before bedtime.

5.   Eat your heaviest meal at the beginning of the day and smaller meals towards the end.

6.   Eat breakfast. Breakfast is your most important meal of the day.

7.   Do not skip meals! A piece of fruit can even be a meal.

8.   Eat something healthy every 3-4 hours.

9.   Use extra virgin olive oil instead of butter or margarine. Note: Many brands of margarine contain a form of MSG.

10.   Eat vegetables and fruits as your main source of foods.

11.   Count your caloric intake. This even includes the foods you taste test or munch on as you are preparing your meals. Remember: Most vegetables are low in calories, but even healthy foods contain calories and natural sugars. So, you still do not want to overdo it by eating too much of any food. Even though the sugars in fruit

are natural sweeteners, and they are healthy, you still do not want to overdo it by eating too many. Until you become familiar with the calorie count of the foods you eat, it's not a bad idea to invest in a calorie-counting book or search the Internet for the caloric content of your food choices. When I am trying to lose weight, eating between 1200-1500 calories a day works best for me.

12.   Take a daily multi-vitamin.

13.   Read food labels.

14.   Eat small food portions. It's best to eat six small meals a day rather than three large ones. This helps to keep your body fueled, which in turn helps to burn calories.

15.   Do not overeat. When you feel full, stop eating. Do not force yourself to continue eating when you are no longer hungry.

16.   Do not continue to eat food that you are not really enjoying. This can often happen when eating food from a restaurant or prepared by someone else. After ordering your food, and you find that you really don't like it, don't continue to eat it. Even though you may think about the money you may have spent for this

food, it is best not to finish eating it. When you do, you end up taking in calories from something that you didn't even enjoy. Also, this increases the amount of your daily caloric intake that could have been avoided or reduced.

17. Determine a reasonable serving size of a food and stick to that portion. For example, your noontime snack may be 12 raw almonds. Place those 12 almonds into a snack pack. Once you eat those 12 almonds, that becomes your allotted amount for the day. As tempting as it may be, do not go back and get more to eat. Don't forget you want to stick to a certain amount of calories for the day and you don't want to use them up by eating extra nuts.

18. It is best not to depend on liquid meal replacement products to reduce your weight. Even if you were to use a liquid drink as a means of weight loss and to replace meals, at some point you are going to have to go back to eating foods. And when you go back to eating foods, you want them to be healthy. So, why not just get into the habit of relying on the healthy foods that your body needs long-term for good nourishment, and that will

help you to lose weight, rather than the short-term meal replacement drinks? However, if you do decide to use a meal replacement drink, be sure to read the label. Even some of those drinks may contain ingredients you may need to avoid.

Try to prepare most of your foods yourself, rather than eating out. You are more aware of the ingredients in the foods you prepare at home than those at a restaurant. However, when eating out, don't hesitate to make special requests. For instance, when ordering a salad, ask to have your salad dressing on the side and with no cheese or croutons. It is best to use oil and vinegar rather than the creamy salad dressings. Request to have your food prepared without butter (or with olive oil) and your vegetables steamed. As you become more familiar with healthy eating, you will understand and know what special requests to make, as well as what foods you should avoid when eating away from home.

Recently, I discovered a restaurant near my neighborhood. After looking at the menu, I inquired as to whether or not they served brown rice. The employee asked me if brown rice was made from wheat. Then the employee informed me that their rice turns brown once they put the soy sauce on it. With those responses, I knew the rice was white and I chose not to eat there. Once again, when eating out at restaurants, ask questions and do not hesitate to make special requests. After all, you want to know and find out as much as you can about the food that is going into your body.

Exercising, particularly strength/resistance training, can cause you to gain muscle. As you gain more muscle, your body burns more fat. As you burn fat, you lose weight. Don't get hung up on weighing yourself on the scales. At times the scales may make it look as if you are not losing weight, when in reality you are. You may be gaining muscle instead of fat, and muscle weighs more than fat. I prefer using a tape measure to track my weight loss more so than getting on a scale. However, I do weigh myself about four times a month.

When you reach a plateau, and you will, don't quit and don't give up. More than likely, when you first start exercising and eating properly, a great amount of your weight will drop. That's because you have introduced a new way of life to your body. But once your body gets used to that change, the weight loss will slow down or even come to a halt. That's when you really have to increase the intensity of your workouts and look again at the foods you are eating. You may also find that you are still eating more food than you are burning up, so you may need to reduce your caloric intake. There is also a possibility that wheat and/or gluten could be the cause of your problems with weight reduction. Gluten is a type of protein, not found in meats, but instead in wheat, oats, barley, rye, and products made from these grains. I have found when I eliminate eating wheat products, which includes bread, my weight drops. You can determine if that's your case by eliminating products containing wheat and/or gluten from your food choices. Wheat and/or gluten may be an ingredient in many of the foods you are eating. Try reducing or eliminating the wheat and/or gluten-containing foods and see what happens. Here is another instance where it is important to read food labels.

Whatever you discover about your food choices, try not to get frustrated with your healthy weight loss plan, because it may take a while. The weight did not come on in one day and it is not going to come off overnight. Anyway, slower is better; quick weight loss is not good on or for your body. Just stick to what you have started, healthy eating and exercising, and it will soon pay off. When you reach your desired weight, continue to eat healthy foods and to incorporate exercising. Eating healthy and exercising should become a way of life — a lifestyle. Not for a temporary period of time just to lose a certain amount of weight, but instead a way of living for the rest of your life. As you implement these lifestyle changes, I am confident you will eventually notice positive changes on the outside of your body, as well as the benefits happening on the inside. Be patient because, as you are becoming a much healthier you, your body is transforming and it is undergoing a worthwhile process of reconstruction.

<u>More Tips for Thought!</u>

- Calories: Take them IN...Burn them OUT!
- Less Eating→ More Moving→ Lose Weight!
- Prayer + Exercise + Healthy Eating = Healthy Weight Loss!!!

Chapter 10

The Many Benefits of Exercising

I can honestly say that I do not have a love affair with exercising. But I do love this life that God has so graciously given to me, and I love living it being healthy and well. So, even though I may not be in love with doing my workouts, I must say that I do love the overall benefits my body gets from exercising.

With so many at-home businesses and all types of jobs being performed just by sitting in front of a computer, the sedentary lifestyle that many of us have grown accustomed to gives us even more reasons why we should exercise. The purchasing of exercise equipment and videos, just looking at them, and allowing them to only occupy space, will get you absolutely no results. Inactivity or lack of exercise can lead to atrophy (decrease of muscle mass-wasting away of muscle) which, in turn, decreases the quality of life. Atrophy of the muscles can expose the body to the attack of so many health problems, some even severe. Helping to prevent atrophy in the body is just one of the many reasons why exercising is so important. Our bodies were designed to be mobile and require movement and physical activity in order for them to reach their peak performance. You've got to get up and move your body...you've got to work your body out! I would also like to point out here that exercising and healthy eating go hand-in-hand. The benefits of healthy eating and the benefits of exercising compliment each other.

As I mentioned in a previous chapter, I started exercising when I clearly heard the Lord tell me that if I didn't start, I was going to die. This was during the period in my life when I was dealing with high cholesterol. My first form of exercise was walking. I went from walking to using machines at the "Y" such as the treadmill, the elliptical trainer, stationary bikes and various types of weight lifting machines. From there I moved to working out with videotapes and DVDs.

One of the first things I had to do when it came to exercising was to get my mind in line with the plan. In doing this, I got my thoughts in the frame of mind that I've got to work out; no ifs, ands, or buts about it. Exercising eventually became just as much a part of my daily routine as brushing my teeth, showering or bathing. I don't know of anyone, to my knowledge, who would go long periods of time without taking this personal time with their body. That is brushing their teeth, showering or bathing. It's not that I am obsessed with exercising, because I am not. Even though I work out five days a week, I don't work out all day long and I take a break from exercising on the weekends. My workouts are anywhere between 30-60 minutes, with the average being about 40 minutes. I have adopted a regular routine of exercising first of all out of a sense of obedience, because of what I told you the Lord said to me back in 1995, and because I have experienced firsthand the benefits from incorporating it into my life. I will admit there are times when I just don't feel like exercising, or I may find a certain exercise to be helpful but yet challenging, so I end up telling myself over and over again, *"I can do all things through Christ which strengthens me."* Before I know it, the workout is over and I have completed a workout that appeared to be very challenging. As I keep reiterating, I want to share with you the things that have helped me to keep healthy and, hopefully, you may find them to be of help to you as well.

I like to use the example of Italian salad dressing when I am teaching on the benefits of exercising. While teaching, as a visual aid, I hold up a bottle of Italian salad dressing. All of the ingredients that help to bring out the best flavor of this dressing are floating on the bottom of the bottle. If you were to just take the bottle and pour the dressing onto your salad without shaking up the ingredients, the taste would be more of oil than anything else, and not very pleasant to the taste buds. However, if you were to shake the bottle and allow all the ingredients to mix together, you can enjoy the full flavor of the dressing. Well, this is how I like to demonstrate one of the benefits of exercising. Our bodies contain many fluids that help to nourish them and keep them running. When we exercise, those fluids are stimulated throughout the body doing their job to take care of the vital organs, muscles, tissues and all the other parts of the body. Just as in the example with the Italian salad dressing, the shaking of the bottle increases the flavor of the dressing, the movement of our body through exercising increases the function of our bodily fluids. This is just one of the many advantages of exercising.

There are more positive benefits to exercising than not. Here is a list of some of the ways in which exercising can be beneficial:

1. Helps to get a healthier and stronger body.

2. Helps to increase the HDL (good cholesterol), and decrease the LDL (bad cholesterol).

3. Helps to lower blood pressure.

4. Helps improve your body composition by burning fat.

5. Helps to build muscle (including the heart, which is also a muscle).

6. Helps to prevent atrophy of the muscles. (The human body has over 600 muscles).

7. Helps to promote bone density. (The human body has 206 bones; 350 at birth).

8. Helps to promote healthy blood sugar levels.

9. Helps to improve blood flow.

10. Helps to boost the immune system.

11. Helps to give the body energy.

12. Helps to boost the metabolism.

13. Helps to improve one's mood. Reduces the chances of depression and reduces stress.

14. Helps to maintain a healthy weight.

15. Helps to improve one's overall health.

16. Helps to make one look and feel younger.

17. Helps to improve posture.

18. Helps to release the chemicals and nutrients into your body that keeps your brain, heart, lungs, cells and other vital parts of your body healthy.

So often we choose to seek the results of what exercising can do for the body externally. In my opinion, the internal benefits far exceed the external. I would therefore suggest that if you feel you've got to focus on one or the other (internal benefits vs. external benefits), focus more on the internal benefits of exercising. As the internal part of the body improves, the external body will have no other choice but to follow suit. You will see a body transformation over time.

I once heard someone say, "If you take care of your body when you are well, your body will take care of you if you get sick." Of course, none of us have a desire to be sick, but if you're injured or if sickness were to attack, by taking care of the body before the injury or sickness, the body will have the ability to heal a lot quicker. Even more so, there would be some health problems that would not even have the chance to attack your body because you have been taking good care of it through proper nutrition and exercising.

Types of Exercises

The different types of exercises are basically: Aerobic, also known as Cardiovascular (Cardio), Strength, which includes Resistance Training, Flexibility and Balance.

Aerobic or Cardiovascular (Cardio)

Aerobic or Cardiovascular (cardio) exercises can be done every day. Some forms of these exercises are:

1. Walking
2. Jogging
3. Stair Stepping
4. Use of Treadmill
5. Use of Elliptical Trainer
6. Biking (Stationary or Regular -- 10-speed, mountain, etc.)
7. Step Aerobics
8. Kickboxing

9. Jumping Rope

10. Hula Hooping

11. Swimming

12. Jumping on a Trampoline

Strength, Resistance, Balance and Flexibility Training

Strength, resistance, balance, or flexibility training can be done in conjunction with the aerobic or cardiovascular (cardio) exercises. When using free weights or weight equipment, such devices should be used every other day, or lower body one day and upper body the next. Your muscles need that time in between your workouts to repair and restore themselves. Some examples of strength, resistance, balance and flexibility training are:

1. Use of free weights. Light weights at five-10 pounds work just fine for me.

2. Use of resistance bands

3. Various types of weight lifting machines

4. Use of a stability ball

5. Pilates

6. Push-ups

7.   Use of your own body weight. This is one of the best forms of strength, resistance, balance and flexibility training.

I made a conscious effort to stay away from free weights and weight lifting machines for a long time because I thought they would cause me to bulk up. But now I realize there are so many great benefits to weight lifting. Strength or resistance training helps to build muscle, which in turn burns fat. It also increases the bone density. As we age, we lose both muscle mass and bone, but strength/resistance training can help improve muscles and bones as well as balance. Flexibility training helps to relieve tension and improves the body's mobility.

I also learned after the age of 50, which I have exceeded, strength or resistance training, balance, and flexibility workouts should become the main focus of my exercise program, while those workouts that jar or put pressure on my joints, such as that in aerobic or cardio exercises, should decrease. Since I now do more strength, resistance, and balancing exercises, I don't do as much when it comes to aerobic or cardio. That's not to say I don't do any aerobic or cardio exercises at all, because I do. Actually, I really like combining strength-type training and cardio into the same workout. This is a form of interval training that can be very effective.

Some Exercising Tips

1.   Block out an hour for each day in which you will exercise. Say for example your exercise hour is 7:00 AM - 8:00 AM on Monday, Wednesday and Friday every week. Even if you do not plan or end up exercising for that full hour, you have still set aside that time between 7:00 AM - 8:00 AM as your designated workout time. As stated earlier, I usually work out for about 40 minutes a day. In this example, if I start at 7:00 AM, then my workout will be over at 7:40. I may decide to call it a day at that point or I may do a few minutes more. On the other hand, within the hour timeframe, I may just decide to work out for 20 minutes and then call it a day. Also, that designated hour may change from day to day. The next day it could be from 8:30-9:30. The point is, I find it to be very helpful in having a designated workout hour each day that I exercise.

My preference is to work out early in the morning. I like to place exercising at the beginning of my day to avoid the possibilities of any other events of the day interfering with the time I set aside for working out. Plus, when it's done early in the morning it's done, it's over with for the day and I can take it off of my *to do* list.

2. Wear comfortable athletic shoes and clothing. You do not have to purchase expensive workout clothes. I bought several pairs of stretchy knit-type leggings (both ankle and knee length) and sport bras from discount stores. When I was working out at the "Y" I would just throw on any old T-shirt from my collection. Most of us have plenty of extra T-shirts, so they can be used to work out in.

Wear ankle supports if you have weak ankles. I wore these for years until my ankles started to get stronger. I preferred the kind that slipped on just like a pair of socks.

Wear two pairs of socks to get additional support and a more cushion-like feeling.

3. Always drink water before, during and after working out.

4. Always warm up before doing any exercise. Always cool down and stretch at the end of each workout. No matter how long or short your workout, it should always include a warm-up and a cool down/stretching. Stretching helps to relax and relieve tension in the muscles. Think of your workout like that of a meal. Your warm-up is your appetizer, the actual workout is your entrée, and your cool down/stretching is your (healthy) dessert.

5. Never hold your breath while working out. Breathe in and out about three counts throughout the workout. Take deep inhales and exhales. The intake of oxygen helps to burn the calories and improves your heart. When using a video or DVD, most of the time the instructor will keep you posted as to when you should inhale and exhale during the routine.

6. Keep your abs (your core section) tight throughout the workout, even when you are not doing abdominal routines. Imagine you are trying to force your belly

button to touch your back; that gives you added strength and helps to improve your posture.

7.   If you exercise using a video or DVD, it is best to view it in its entirety before doing the actual workout. This way you will have a better idea of what to expect once you are ready to do the exercise routine.

8.   When exercising to a video or DVD, count as the routine is being performed. This helps you to continue to breathe and not hold your breath. Usually routines on videos or DVDs are in counts of eight, 10, 12 or 16. I found it's best to keep up with my own counting because some instructors on the video or DVD will have fewer counts of the exercise on one side of the body than the other. For example, they may do eight leg lifts on the right side and do the same leg lift on the left side and give it 12 counts. You want the exact number of counts on each side when doing the same exercise. By keeping track of your own count, not only will it help to remind you to keep breathing, but you will know if you need to do more or less of the routine than what is instructed on the video or DVD.

9.   When doing exercises to a DVD or video, pay attention to the side the instructor is telling you to work out on. There are those instructors, the kind I prefer, who will instruct you to move in the direction they want you to go in while you are facing the television. In other words, if they want you to work out your left side, they will say your left, or if they want you on your right side they will say right. On the other hand, some instructors will tell you to do a particular exercise on your right side. It may be their right side, but it's your left. Or they may tell you to do a routine on your left side when it is in fact your right but their left. During the workout, this can become just as confusing as it sounds. So, whether the fitness instructor tells you to make your move on your right side or your left side, it's always a good idea to perform the exercise in the same direction the instructor and/or the DVD or video participants are performing it as you face the television screen. By doing this, it helps you to keep up with the routine and reduces the possibility of any confusion as to which side you should be working out on.

10. Stay focused on your workout. Avoid distractions such as thinking about work, what you are going to wear next week, what you are going to eat when you finish working out, etc. Avoid an excessive amount of talking If your telephone rings, let the voicemail take your messages. You want to give your workout as much of your undivided attention as you possibly can.

11. It is best to work out on an empty stomach or at least an hour after you have eaten. Otherwise, the body is not only concentrating on the exercise, but on digesting the food as well. Exercising is most beneficial when your body only has the exercise to deal with. Aside from water, I do not put anything else into my body until I have completed my exercise for the day.

12. As you conquer doing low impact workouts for about 10 to 20 minutes, three times a week, gradually work towards increasing your intensity, minutes, and the number of workout days per week.

13. About every eight to 12 weeks change your exercise routine. After this period of time, your body will get accustomed to the routine and you will reach a plateau. You will reach a point where your body will not want

to cooperate with your workout. It will be as if it's telling you, *"Oh, I see now what you are trying to do to me, so I am not going to cooperate. I am not going to budge."* This is where you need to take control of your body by showing it what you want it to do, not it showing you. Changing your workout routine and increasing your intensity will help to break through that plateau. You will need to start playing tricks on your body by introducing it to something that it has not yet experienced. Then when it becomes familiar with that routine, change up — trick it again, by challenging it with something else different. This *tricking* cycle will go on and on in order to get your body to continue to cooperate. After a while, you can even go back to routines that you have done in the past, because your body will have forgotten about them. By the time it remembers and goes back to being uncooperative, you can once again trick it by changing your workout.

Changing up your routines also allows you to force yourself to do more advanced and/or challenging exercises. Periodically, you really do want to challenge yourself with your workouts and go beyond your level of comfort.

14.   When doing certain exercises, such as squats or lunges, always keep your knees soft (bent) as you are performing the routine. If you are doing an exercise where your entire leg needs to be completely straight, such as a side leg lift, then it's all right not to bend your leg during the routine.

Never jerk or snap your knee into position.

Avoid putting pressure on your knee(s) even when doing any type of stretching. I really believe the knee injury that I mentioned in a previous chapter was partly due to exercising improperly. I would place my hand on the side of my knee, instead of on my thigh or calf, and hold a side stretch. I was putting too much pressure on my knee and in time, I paid for it.

As a side note, never use your knee as a piece of equipment. For example, if you are trying to move some furniture, do not use your knee(s) to help in moving or pushing it. You can possibly cause injury to your knee(s) that could easily have been prevented.

15. Sweat! This helps to remove toxins from your body. Try not to use a fan, because this only decreases the sweat that would otherwise excrete from your body.

16. It is very common and easy to allow tension in your neck, but try to keep your neck relaxed during your workout.

17. If you have an injury or sprain a muscle, don't use that particular part of the body until it is healed. For example, I sprained my tricep in my left arm. I had to stop doing strength training for my arms until that muscle healed. As long as I was continuing to strength train and lift weights, it was not healing. When I stopped with the strength and weight training, the muscle healed so much quicker. It did not stop me, for there was no need to, from working out the other parts of my body during this time of healing.

18. If you start feeling dizzy or lightheaded while working out, stop, take a break or discontinue the workout until

these feelings subside. It is very important to listen to your body in this instance.

19.   While working out, I like to monitor my heart with the use of a heart monitor. This enables me to keep better track of my target heart rate during my workout. You can also measure your target heart rate by taking the beats of your pulse periodically as you are working out. This requires using one set of fingers, placing them on the opposite wrist or on the neck, and counting the beats. My preference is to use a heart rate monitor set with the strap that goes around the chest and a wristwatch that can be easily viewed while working out. To me, the heart rate monitor sets around $25 work just as well as the more expensive ones.

As you exercise, you want to stay within 50 to 75 percent of your maximum heart rate. This range is called your target heart rate zone. When starting an exercise program, aim at the lowest range of your target zone (50 percent) during the first few weeks. Gradually build up to the higher number of your target zone (75 percent). After six months or more of regular exercise, you may be able to exercise comfortably at up to 85 percent of your maximum heart rate. However, you don't have to exercise that hard to stay in shape.

To help burn fat, you want to maintain your workout within your target heart rate zone. Your target heart rate is the number of times your heart beats per minute. The following is an example of a calculation of a target heart rate zone for someone who is 53 years:

220-53 (age) =167 (220 minus your age)

Minimum- 167 x 50 percent = 84

Maximum- 167 x 75 percent = 125

Maximum- (After six months of regular exercise) 167 x 85 percent =142

In this example, at age 53, the target heart rate zone during exercise is 84 to125. Once this 53-year-old becomes advanced, the target heart rate zone is 84 to142.

Eliminate Excuses

There are numerous excuses as to why people choose not to exercise. Here are just a few of them, along with my response:

Excuse #1: Lack of time due to work and/or family commitments.

Response: We have to make time. We can find time to do anything that we really want to do. Even if it means getting up a little earlier, going to bed earlier so you can get up earlier, cutting out some television, computer or telephone talking time.

Excuse #2: Cost of equipment or gym membership is way too expensive.

Response: Walking, videotapes, DVDs, and free weights are relatively inexpensive compared to a gym membership. If you don't want to invest in free weights, canned foods can be used instead. With the use of the Internet, there are hundreds of workout programs you can learn. There are also many television networks that broadcast exercise programs. Once you learn how and what to do, you can make up your own exercise routines. You can also check with your local library and see what type of exercise DVDs or videos they have that you can check out.

Excuse #3: There are no workout facilities near my home.

Response: Work out at home.

Excuse #4: I get bored with exercising.

Response: Switch up your workouts. Have a variety of different exercise videos or DVDs. Think about the benefits, because they truly outweigh the boredom.

Excuse #5: I can't work out by myself, or I don't like working out alone.

Response: Join some type of exercise class or find yourself a workout buddy if you can. However, there will come a point in time when you can no longer depend on someone else for your workout routine. Even with a workout buddy, there are going to be days when you will want to work out and your buddy will not.

It is best not to become so dependent on others to the extent that they determine whether or not you work out. A workout partner is good if you are the type that needs one, but learn to be independent when it comes to exercising. Eventually, it should become imperative for you to realize that you and only you alone can do this for yourself...not anyone else. When it comes to working out, one is not a lonely number!

Stay Motivated

1. Remember, your body is the temple of God and you want to keep it in good condition for Him. That alone should be a motivator. When working out, I sometimes have to quote Scriptures to make it through the workout. The one I quote the most is, as previously mentioned, *"I can do all things through Christ which strengthens me."*

2. Be **consistent** with exercising. Keep at it over and over and over again on a regular basis. Once you make exercising a habit, it will be just like any other habit — hard to break.

3. Be **committed** to exercising. Make it just as much a part of your life as brushing your teeth. If you miss any of your time or days you have carved out for exercising, don't give up — just pick up and start again.

4. Constantly **challenge** yourself with different and even more intense workouts. When you get out of your comfort zone, it helps to take your exercise routine to another level.

Children and Exercise

Without a change, it is my understanding that today's younger generation is predicted to be the first generation to die before their previous generation. Improper eating and lack of exercise will play a major role in this prediction. Children today are exposed to so much that inhibits mobility and provides convenience, such as: video games, remote controls, vending machines, and no real physical education or activity in their schools. Get your children, grandchildren, nieces, nephews, cousins, friend's kids, everyone you possibly can into exercising. We don't want to see this generation of children suffer with sicknesses and diseases when we can do something to help prevent it from happening. If we as parents and as adults do not encourage exercising, then our children are not going to be enthused about it either. Let your children see you exercising, discuss it with them, and do some exercises together. Let's do our part to help motivate our children for now, and for the future of their good health.

Get a Check-up

Before you or your child start a workout routine, please see your doctor to make sure you and/or your child are physically able to perform regular exercise. You would not want to experience an adverse reaction to exercising that may possibly result in it aggravating or triggering a medical condition that you were totally unaware of, and that could have been treated beforehand

Chapter 11

Other Health-Related Topics

<u>Everyday Practices</u>

Licking Stamps & Envelopes

Please try to avoid licking stamps and envelopes. Most stamps now contain their own adhesive, so they don't require moisture like they have in the past. But just in case you run across some stickers or some other type of stamp that requires moistening, use water instead of placing them on your tongue. The same goes for envelopes. There was a time when I would lick envelopes, and I noticed shortly after doing so, I would get a headache. It soon occurred to me that the glue on the envelope was not designed to be eaten. Its purpose was to seal the envelope, not for me to consume. I then invested in some glue sticks. I always keep some on hand. I even purchased some for each of my family members to carry in their Bible cases, to use whenever they need to seal the tithes and offering envelopes. The investment into the glue sticks certainly beats licking and eating something that has absolutely no business in our bodies.

Hand Washing

It is so important to thoroughly wash your hands. Wash them when you go to the bathroom, when you comb your hair, when you blow your nose...wash your hands. I truly believe that so many illnesses could be avoided simply by keeping your hands clean.

When in a restaurant, I often see people handle a menu and then touch their food. I realize we have no control over, and have no idea, what goes on in the kitchen as our food is being prepared, but we can control those things that we do see. When we touch a menu, we have no clue as to who else touched it or where their hands have been. Some people will not wash their hands after touching different parts of their body if their life depended on it. After touching their different body parts, the germs on their hands are then transferred to the menu. If we don't wash our hands after handling the menu, and later touch our food, we invite so many of those germs to enter into our bodies.

Another thing that I often observe in restaurants is, after handling the menu, a person takes a lemon, squeezes the juice into the glass and then throws the lemon rind into the drink. There go all the germs from the menu and from the lemon rind, into the drink and then into the person's body.

Even if we do not handle a menu, there are germs on our cars' steering wheels, on door handles, and even our very own cell phones are loaded with germs. I am not saying we can live in a totally germ-free world, but there are things we can do to cut down on the possibility of germs invading our systems. Even when I am at home cooking or eating, and I stop to answer the telephone or touch the television remote control, I wash my hands before I go back to preparing or eating my meal. Our very own hands can carry so many germs. With those germs on our hands, every time we touch our face, put our fingers in the corners of our eyes, in our mouths, or on the food we eat, we ingest those germs.

It is very important to teach children about the importance of washing their hands as well. Recently, I visited an elementary school and there was a sign in the restroom encouraging its (the restroom's) visitors to wash their hands. The sign suggested singing a verse of *Old McDonald Had a Farm* as you are washing your hands. The completion of that verse would allow for a good hand washing. I thought that was a cute way for kids, as well as adults, to know how long it would take to give their hands a good washing. If you don't want to sing, just count out 20 seconds.

In order to get a thorough washing, you want the water to be as hot as you can possibly stand it. Even though I prefer good old soap and water, for those times when you don't have water readily available, use a hand sanitizer. Keep some in your car, in your purse, wallet, computer case, or wherever, but just always have some on hand.

Many of the stores are now providing sanitized wipes so that you can wipe off the handle of the shopping cart when you enter the store. Since these sanitizers are only used occasionally, take advantage of the wipes — use them whenever they are available. Here again, you have no idea where all of those hands have been that have touched the cart. Sometimes we will leave that same store, after handling the cart and money (which, by the way, is loaded with germs) and open one of the items we just purchased because hunger has hit and we want a quick snack. This is where the hand sanitizer will definitely come in handy.

When checking out at a store, if you have a cashier who likes to use their spit to open the plastic bag that they are putting your items into, you can ask them in a polite manner not to lick their fingers and then touch your bags. When I find them licking their fingers when packing my bags, I will usually say something like, "Do you mind not licking your fingers?" Or if I see a wet sponge on the counter I'll say, "Would you be so kind and use the wet sponge to pack my bags?" At one store, the cashier has named me "The no lick lady!" On one occasion, when I politely asked the cashier not to lick her fingers, she told me, "I'm not touching the part you will be touching!" She said that as if it really made a difference. I still let her know I would appreciate her not licking her fingers to pack my bags. There is no reason to be shy about asking people to keep their spit to themselves. You did not come to the store to purchase their spit, and you should not have to take it home with your merchandise.

I know most people mean well when they touch a baby's hand, but that is so unfair to the baby. Babies are constantly putting their hands in their faces, touching their eyes and putting their hands into their mouths. Then along comes an adult or an older child, "Oh, she/he is so precious," and grabs the baby's hand or rubs the baby's face. Babies can be admired without touching their hand(s) or stroking their face. A baby's immune system is so delicate and does not need to be subjected to the many germs his/her admirers carry on their hands.

Another thing, when you go to the doctor or dentist, or any health care provider, don't be afraid or hesitant to ask them to wash their hands before they start to examine you. Many health care providers do wash their hands, but there are also some who do not. They will work on patient after patient and never wash their hands. You have no idea what the previous patient(s) had, so please don't be bashful in requesting a hand washing before you are touched.

Here's a side note, but a true story, that I want to share that I saw with my own eyes at a five-star hotel. Phil and I were on vacation and stayed in this really exclusive hotel. Phil had gone out to play golf and I was just resting in the room. When the housekeeper came to clean the room, I informed her that we did not have any clean glasses. She went out into the hall, took dirty glasses that had been placed on the bottom of her cart, and commenced to wiping them off, inside and out, with the same rag she had just cleaned the bathroom with. She then held each glass up to the light, wiped them a couple more times until they were shining like new money. I expressed my dissatisfaction to her in doing this, but from that day to this, I refuse to drink out of hotel glasses. Also, it reminded me that everything that shines isn't always clean!

Holding Handrails

As I was growing up, my mother would always remind me to hold onto handrails when going up and down stairs. Back in 2008, while walking on a college campus, as Phil and I were going down some stairs, the heel of my shoe got caught between a brick and I fell. Everything I was carrying commenced to flying in different directions. As my husband was helping me up off of the ground, I could hear my mother's voice reminding me to hold on to the handrail. I was blessed to have only sprung my left ankle. But you know what? From then on, I started holding onto handrails every time I go up and down stairs. I do this even in my own home. We all may possibly know of someone or even a number of people who have sustained serious falls down stairs, oftentimes even in their own homes. Some of those falls ended up causing permanent injuries or in some cases, even death. So my advice here is to hold onto those rails no matter how long or short of a distance you are going up or down the stairs. The handrails were placed there for a reason, for us to hold on to.

Driving and Cell Phone Usage/Car Maintenance

I recently saw a television show where families had lost loved ones due to someone talking or texting while driving. During this show, there were some individuals who caused the accidents and lived to talk about it. They were pleading with others not to text or talk on cell phones while driving. They were feeling so awful and remorseful because they had caused the death of another person due to the split second they decided to use their cell phones. There were also doctors on this program who said the brain cannot completely focus on driving as well as texting or talking on the phone at the same time. Furthermore, a person's ability to react and respond is decreased. The doctors went on to say, even if a person uses an earpiece, talking and/or texting while driving is equivalent to someone driving drunk. That story quickly got my attention and changed my behavior when it comes to the use of my cell phone while driving.

I would venture to say the same holds true with searching for CDs or changing them while driving or any other things that can be a distraction. Recently, while riding with Phil on the interstate, I saw a man with his cell phone propped up against his shoulder and he was flipping through papers he had on top of his steering wheel as if the steering wheel was a desk in his office. He was doing all of this while driving about 60 miles per hour. I thought I had seen it all when it came to the unsafe things people do while driving, but I think this one topped them all.

Talking, texting, changing CDs, reading or any other distraction, can be hazardous to your life or the life of someone else. If any of these activities need to be conducted while driving, please pull off to the side of the road so that you will not be distracted from driving, or stand the chance of putting your life or the lives of others in harm's way. On the other hand, if you happen to observe someone conducting any of these activities while you are driving, it is best to get as far away from them as soon as you possibly can.

When driving, be sure not to exceed the speed limit. Pay attention to the speed limit signs and adhere to them. Speeding can result in accidents that may have lasting and harmful affects on you as well as others.

Since the vast majority of us operate motor vehicles on a daily or a regular basis, it is to our benefit to keep them in tip-top shape. On January 24, 2009, I had an experience with my automobile that I pray will never happen again. While driving my car on the interstate during a snowstorm and in blizzard-like conditions, I lost complete control of my automobile. My car started to spin out of control and I could not do or say anything except JESUS. Even though I was headed north on the interstate, when my car stopped spinning, I was facing south. After spinning for what seemed like eternity, my car came to a complete stop. I was so terrified but yet so thankful that I was not hurt and neither was anyone else. I later learned that the rear tires on my car were practically bald. There was very little traction left on the tires and I was completely unaware of it. Phil and I had not been taking care of nor paying attention to my vehicle like we should have, and it could have possibly cost me my life or the life of someone else.

I share this as a reminder as to how important it is to keep the maintenance up on our automobiles. We cannot just ride around in our cars, not take good care of them, and expect them to continue to operate to their fullest potential. Without proper care of our vehicles, eventually something is bound to go wrong.

So, please keep your vehicles properly serviced; this includes tire checks. Also, when driving a motor vehicle, please give it your undivided attention by not talking on your cell phone (even with an earpiece), texting or doing anything else that may cause a distraction. And, do not exceed the speed limit when driving. The possible detrimental consequences of any of these things (driving around in a vehicle that's not well maintained, a chit-chat or sending a typed message while operating a motor vehicle, or speeding) is definitely not worth it.

Snow Removal

If you live in a region that gets snow, like I do, and you are over the age of 50, you should avoid the task of snow removal. This includes removing snow using either a snow shovel or a snow blower. There have been cases of people over the age of 50 who were in the best of health, dying from heart attacks as a result of conducting the task of removing snow. It has been found that this activity can over-stress the heart. Coupled with that and the change in body temperature that takes place, this plays a major role in the attack that can possibly take place on the heart. As a result, it has been recommended that anyone over the age of 50 should not engage in the removal of snow. Even if you are not over the age of 50, but you have certain health issues, like heart-related conditions, or obesity, it's probably a good idea for you to avoid the task of snow removal as well. I know that there are times when you can't even get out of your driveway because of the amount of snow that has accumulated, but if need be, hire someone, even some kids, to remove it for you. And if you don't really have to go anywhere, stay in the house if you can't get out. One thing for sure, it won't be long before the snow will melt on its own. It's definitely not worth the risk you place on yourself that's associated with removing snow either by shoveling or the use of a snow blower. After all, wouldn't paying someone or just waiting until it melts on its own be a better alternative to a heart attack? This is just something else to think about and to take into consideration.

Household Products

As I discussed earlier, if foods contain ingredients that you can't pronounce, then it does the body good not to eat them. Well, the same goes for household products. If they contain words you cannot pronounce, then it does not help the body to use them. When we use bleach (even though that's a word we can pronounce), window/glass cleaners, bathroom cleaners, oven cleaners, etc., our bodies are taking in the chemicals they contain. We can breathe them into our systems and they can get into our bodies by way of our skin or even through our eyes.

To avoid these harmful chemicals, what I started doing was using white vinegar and baking soda as cleaning agents. Both vinegar and baking soda are ingredients that are safe if inhaled or consumed by the body. As a window/glass cleaner, in a spray bottle, I fill about three-fourths of the bottle with white vinegar and one-fourth of it with water. This combination does an excellent job on cleaning mirrors, glass table tops and windows, and I am not inhaling the fumes that I used to get while using those other products loaded with all sorts of chemicals. I use baking soda for those jobs where I used to use cleanser, and it gets the job done too. I get great results when cleaning some places, like the toilet, by using a combination of white vinegar and baking soda.

Think about insect sprays. If they are powerful enough to kill insects, what could they possibly be doing to the insides of our bodies as we inhale those fumes? Just a thought! What about air fresheners that we spray into the air, and how we breathe in those fumes? Keep in mind, whatever we inhale and whatever goes onto our skin also enters the body and could very well be playing a role in damaging it. I realize there are some things that we do not have any control over when it comes to what we inhale or what the outside of our bodies are exposed to, but there are things that we do have control over. There are insect sprays, air fresheners, and other household products you can use that do not contain the chemicals that can be harmful to your health. What I am suggesting here is to be aware of what chemicals you inhale, what you put on your skin, and the types of everyday ingredients (even those contained in perfumes, colognes, lotions, etc.) that you expose your body to.

On two separate occasions, I was experiencing some type of discomfort on my body and the doctor could not determine the problem. One was a female problem and the other was an irritation on my chest. In each instance, after having a number of tests conducted and being prescribed creams that did not work (even one costing $113 -- thank God for insurance), I discovered the female problem was caused by the bath soap I was using, and the irritation on my chest by the laundry detergent. Once I changed bath soap and later laundry detergent, the problems went away. This is an example of how we can sometimes be misdiagnosed and prescribed unnecessary medication for something that may only require a simple change. In addition, it shows how some ordinary household products can irritate the body and be the cause of some of our health issues.

Keeping Surroundings Tidy

We may not often think of it in this context, but untidy surroundings can be stress-inducers. For many years, I found it very difficult to keep my house tidy. It was not nasty, but it was extremely cluttered. I did not like the way it looked, yet I felt like there was nothing I could really do about it because this was just how I was. At times, it would be rather embarrassing when someone would drop by the house. My body would get into fast gear to at least make the house half-way presentable before they arrived. Clothes that I had recently worn and/or those that had been washed would be scattered here and there. Throwing and hiding things in the closet and waiting until a later day and time to wash dishes had become the norm. This was a way of living that went on for many years in my life, and it was rather stressful to say the least. Until one day the change started.

Phil and I had prayed and asked the Lord for our dream home. We believed we were going to get it and we wanted it to be in Ohio, my home state. We did not know when and we did not even know exactly where in Ohio it was going to be. We just believed it was coming. We went as far as putting the layout of our home on paper and listing all the specifics we wanted it to include. (Habakkuk 2:2-3 — *"And the LORD answered me, and said, Write the vision, and make it plain upon tables, that he may run that readeth it. For the vision is yet for an appointed time, but at the end it shall speak, and not lie: though it tarry, wait for it; because it will surely come, it will not tarry."*)

We had purchased a coffee table, a lamp and one end table for our family room in Birmingham. The family room was not big enough for two end tables. But several months later, I told Phil we needed to go back to the furniture store and purchase another lamp and end table, because one day we would have a family room big enough to accommodate them. We did just that and stored them in a spare bedroom for years.

One day I said, "Lord, I believe You are going to bless us with our dream home, but I need Your help in knowing how to keep a tidy house. I need Your help because I really don't know what to do or how to do it. I want our house to represent You in the spirit of excellence." This may seem like a ridiculous prayer, but God knew the sincerity of my heart. I was serious. Shortly after that time, Phil and I moved to a duplex home in Broken Arrow, Oklahoma. The home was much smaller than what we had while we were living in Birmingham. But this was the home where the Lord started teaching and showing me about tidiness. He began to show me simple things like when you are finished with something, put it back were it belongs. Everything should have its proper place in the home and that is where it should reside. Otherwise, if you don't put it back, then stuff will start to pile up and then you will have clutter all over again.

Here's another one. When you take off your clothes hang them up. That sounds like a no-brainer, but for years I would leave my clothes at the foot of the bed or in a chair, and I would hang them up tomorrow. Well, tomorrow would never come, as far as hanging up my clothes, so those piles at the foot of the bed and in the chair only got higher and higher. When I would wash clothes, instead of folding them up and putting them away, they would remain in the laundry basket and we would just pick them out of the basket as needed. How much simpler and less cluttered it would have been to just fold the clothes up as they were taken out of the dryer. Now, as I strive to be more disciplined with keeping the house tidy, the clothes are folded and put away when they come out of the dryer.

Another simple tidbit that was revealed to me was picking up lint off of the carpeting. There could be four or five pieces of lint, thread, or whatever, lying on the floor, which makes the carpet look like it needs to be vacuumed. Sure, at some point the carpet will need a good vacuum cleaning, but just picking up those four or five pieces of lint, thread, or whatever, off the carpet can give it a freshly vacuumed look.

As I began to do the different things the Lord was showing me, keeping the house tidy became easier and easier. While we were living in Oklahoma, I remember a friend of ours who came to visit saying, "Your house is so neat and clean!" My, how good those words sounded in my ears. I had never in my life had anyone say that to me (because they did not have any reason to). I thanked the Lord and realized the discipline the Lord was teaching me was just a rehearsal for our future dream home.

Well, in May 2008, we officially moved into our faith/dream home. We were able to put that additional lamp and end table in it as well. And keeping an untidy house has so far been a thing of the past. I am not claiming to be a perfect housekeeper, because I am not, but I can say that I do not keep house anywhere near the way I used to. Since moving into our home, we have had countless numbers of compliments on how neat, clean and tidy our home is. I am very quick to tell people that it has not always been this way for me. I had to seek the Lord's help, and He delivered me from being an untidy housekeeper and taught me what to do to be a tidy one.

Some may be asking: What does this have to do with a healthy lifestyle? It plays its part in the mix. It's like when you get a dirty car all cleaned and freshened up, it seems to ride better. Or when you put clean linen on the bed, the bed feels so refreshing. You see, when your surroundings are in order, it helps you to feel good about yourself. Well, at least it does for me. I no longer get that added pressure of knowing I need to clean up or straighten up, and wishing it would happen on its own. Straightening up, picking up, and cleaning up as we go, makes it so much easier to keep our surroundings tidy. This discipline the Lord taught me does not even require a lot of hard work or long hours of cleaning. It's amazing how this works, and it's just one less thing to possibly get stressed out about.

If God answers simple prayers such as being a better housekeeper and finding that dream home, He certainly will answer your prayers if you desire to live a healthier lifestyle. Why? It's because your body and your life are more valuable and of greater importance to Him.

Body Maintenance

Overcoming Food Addictions

Most of us may not want to admit it, but we can in fact be addicted to food just like some people are addicted to drugs, alcohol, and smoking. For those who are addicted to these damaging substances, one of the first steps in being delivered from such addictions is to admit that they are in fact an addict. The same thing holds true for food addicts. When individuals sincerely admit and acknowledge that they are addicted to the wrong kinds of foods, or even the consumption of too much food, they have accomplished one of the first steps to deliverance from food addiction. Alcoholics, drug addicts, smokers and food addicts all have some things in common. They are doing those things to their bodies that can destroy their God-given temples and cause their bodies to age prematurely. Just as with a drug addict, a smoker, or an alcoholic, it's not uncommon for a food addict to deny there is a problem and that help is needed. But once they come clean and honest with themselves, they can move towards healing and deliverance from such an addiction.

I will admit I once had food addictions. These addictions are what caused me to have high cholesterol and some other health issues that I shared earlier. It was not until I took control of the poor eating habits and incorporated a healthy lifestyle that I even realized I had food addictions. The question I eventually asked myself was, *"Do you love this bad food more than you love your life, or do you love your life more than you love the bad food?"* Of course my response was I love my life more than I love the bad food. With that being the case, I needed to act like it. It was one thing for me to say I loved life more than unhealthy food, but it was another to exhibit it. My actions certainly had to speak louder than my words, so I decided to take the necessary steps to prove to myself and to show my Lord my appreciation for my body. This meant I could no longer abuse it with unhealthy foods, and I had to take better care of it.

So, if you have food addictions, there is nothing wrong with admitting to it. Actually, that's a good thing. If you acknowledge the addiction and really want to take positive actions towards dealing with it, you will then open the door to overcoming one of your biggest obstacles — from (possibly) that of denial to that of admission. You can then start on the road of incorporating and living a healthier lifestyle.

The Importance of Drinking Water

I cannot emphasize enough the importance of drinking water. Water helps to keep the body's fluids running properly. It aids in strengthening the muscles, helps to lubricate the joints and keeps the body's organs functioning properly. It rids the body of toxins and helps to flush out of the body those things that may otherwise harm it. It helps to improve the skin. And the list goes on and on.

The amount of ounces of water you take in on a daily basis should be equivalent to half your body weight. If you weigh 200 pounds, then you should drink 100 ounces of water per day. If you find that too difficult to do initially, start off with eight glasses a day, but eventually you want to consume half your body weight. The best way I have found for me to get in my daily amount of water is to fill up a glass pitcher equivalent to half my body weight, and pour from that pitcher throughout the day. I either pour water from it into a glass, or pour it into a smaller glass water bottle. Taking water with me wherever I go is also very helpful. It allows me to sip/drink water throughout the day. Before I know it, I have gotten in my desired daily amount.

The water mixed with tea, coffee, or whatever other liquid you may drink, does not count as drinking water. I am talking about plain old water with nothing added to it except perhaps juice from a fresh lemon.

Once again, we have something here that God made for our consumption — WATER! Water is the best liquid you can place into your body. It is very good for you and it provides many health benefits. If you don't like water or have not been drinking it, hopefully the fact that it is good for you and that it provides many health benefits will be a motivator to start including it in your daily liquid intake.

Note: If you happen to drink water from a plastic bottle, do not drink it after it has been left in a car and gotten warm or hot. Even when the bottle is not hot, some plastics have a tendency to leach toxins into the water and may cause serious harm to your body. What I have chosen to do is to avoid drinking from plastic water bottles or plastic containers altogether. Even though there are certain types of plastics that don't leach chemicals, glass containers are my first choice and stainless steel is second. By the way, hazardous plastic is also found in the lining of some of the cans used for canned foods. I suggest doing an Internet search to get more information on the leaching of chemicals from plastic bottles, the dangers of plastic water bottles and the dangers of plastic linings in canned foods.

Taking Nutritional Supplements

Unfortunately, even the healthiest of foods lose some of their nutritional value. This can be as a result of long storage life, from the way it was grown or whatever. That is why I have found it so important to take supplements. My daily supplementation currently includes: a good multi-vitamin, vitamin C, calcium containing magnesium and vitamin D, a vegetable supplement, vitamin B-12 -sublingual- (taken under the tongue), resveratrol, lutein, hyaluronic acid with collagen, and MSM, bilberry, fish oil, a good probiotic, the spice turmeric and vitamin D3 (often referred to as the miracle vitamin).

Turmeric helps to keep the inflammation down in the body and helps to reduce aches and pains in the joints. As a preventive measure, I take a teaspoon with about six to eight ounces of water followed by another six to eight ounces of plain water. Even though I prefer the actual spice, and can use it as an ingredient to season my food, turmeric is also available in capsule form.

Vitamin D is often referred to as the miracle vitamin because of the ways in which it can help with so many health problems. Vitamin D naturally comes from the sun. In about 30 minutes of sunshine, an average person can get about 10,000 IUs (International Units) of vitamin D. (Be sure to wear sunscreen if you are exposed to the sun for more than 10 minutes). I once heard a true story of a lady who had been diagnosed with cancer. She said the Lord told her to sit by the window in her house and take in the sunshine. She faithfully did what the Lord told her and was eventually healed.

I would highly recommend you looking into the many benefits of vitamin D, including vitamin D-3. You may find it may be very helpful for you to supplement this vitamin as well.

Garlic is also good to help reduce levels of high blood pressure or high cholesterol. Fresh garlic cloves can be swallowed (it's best to cut it up) with a glass of water or it can be taken in pill or capsule form.

Depending on your individual needs, you may find that you may need more or less than what I take, but either way, I believe it's a good idea to take nutritional supplements of some kind. If you are dealing with a particular aliment and are taking supplements to relieve it, be patient. Oftentimes supplements do not work as quickly as perhaps medication, but just give it time before giving up its use.

If you are on any kind of medication and are taking supplements, you should take the medication and supplements at least two hours apart from each other. This helps to cut down on the possibility of one group of ingredients interfering with the effectiveness of the other. With the exception of vitamin D and magnesium, in order to get the most of its absorption when taking a calcium supplement, it is best to take it separately from any other supplements. Also, the body only absorbs up to 500 milligrams of calcium at a time. If you are taking more than that amount per day, then it is best to take the dosages separately so that you can reap the benefits of the total amount you are taking in a day. For instance, if you are taking 1,000 milligrams of calcium a day, take 500 milligrams in the afternoon and 500 milligrams later in the evening.

If a supplement's directions state it should be taken with a meal, then it is best to take it with food. If it says you can take it with or without food, then it can be taken on a full or an empty stomach. To get the best out of your supplements, be sure to follow the directions on how they should be taken.

- First and foremost, you want to obtain your nutrients from the foods you eat. Supplements should be taken in addition to food, not instead of food.

- Be sure to find a good multi-vitamin for your children. Children need to be on good nutritional supplements as well.

- Be sure to read the labels, because you want to avoid those nutritional supplements containing MSG or sugar.

- Taking good nutritional supplements is a great companion to healthy eating.

- Be sure to check with your professional health care provider before you or your child/children take any nutritional supplements.

Medication(s)

As you probably know by now, I am not one to readily take medication, however I do believe if you have a health issue that has gotten out of control and your doctor has prescribed medication, then you should take it. For example, if your blood pressure is extremely high, and medication is recommended, then you should take it, for it may in fact save your life. I still believe, however, that incorporating a healthy lifestyle could very well prevent the attack of many health issues before they even become a problem. Also, just because you are on medication, that does not mean that's an invitation to eat unhealthy or not to exercise. Someone once told me, because they were on medication for high cholesterol, they ate unhealthy and relied on the medication to keep them healthy. That, of course, is not the attitude to take at all. Even when you are on medication, you should still eat right and exercise. Doing so could possibly help you to get off the medication. Be sure to discuss with your doctor any supplements you are taking, or want to take, along with your medication.

Please Note: It has been reported that grapefruit can interfere with certain medications. If you are on medication and eat grapefruit or drink its juice, please check with your doctor to see if this includes the medication(s) you are on. You can search the Internet for this information as well, but still be sure to consult with your doctor. Aside from the interference with certain medications, grapefruit, just like fruits in general, has so many benefits including improving bone health. So if you are not on any of the medications in question, take advantage of the great nutrients contained in grapefruit.

Annual Physical Examinations

It is so important to make sure that we get physical examinations. Even if we are not having any physical problems, we should get our bodies checked out by a professional health care provider. My preference is to have an annual physical.

There are many people who do not care to or want to go to the doctor, but yet they make every effort to take care of the maintenance on their motor vehicles. They take their vehicle to the urgent car care hospital for a tune-up, an oil change and/or just for a general inspection. Shouldn't we give our temples even more care and attention than our motor vehicles? I would think so. There are those who may say they don't have the money to get an annual physical exam, but if their cars break down, every effort is made, and somehow accomplished, to get the funds to repair that vehicle.

If you were to find you are faced with needing additional funds, after whatever the government provides in the form of health care, you can start putting aside a little bit of extra money every month to save for any possible added medical expenses in the future. You may be surprised at the amount of money you will have just by saving a little bit of it over an extended period of time. The additional amount of money it may cost you, over and above what the government has to offer with health care, could very well reduce the cost of any possible health problem(s) detected, treated or prevented altogether, as a result of having a thorough annual (or regular) physical examination.

Even though I may have refused some surgeries, I do believe certain tests and screenings should be conducted, such as: cholesterol test, blood pressure check, blood sugar screening, prostate screening (men), pap smear (women), a colonoscopy, the checking of vitamin D, B-12, potassium and calcium levels, just to name a few. High blood pressure and high cholesterol are not always identified by symptoms like some other medical conditions. That is why they are often referred to as the silent killers. Blood pressure and cholesterol levels can be determined by being checked and screened. If they go undetected, they can eventually cause major health problems or even death.

There may be times when your doctor may not suggest certain tests or screenings, so you will have to take charge and request them yourself. You should become familiar with those areas of your body you should have checked, and when. For example, at age 50 (age 40 if there's a family history of polyps or colon cancer), it is recommended to have a colonoscopy at least every 10 years. Some doctors even recommend every five years, and even more frequently if polyps are ever detected. During a colonoscopy, if polyps are found they can be removed, and there goes the chance of them possibly turning into cancer. However, it has been stated by the medical profession that if the polyps are not detected and not removed, they can eventually turn into cancer in the colon.

During a recent colonoscopy that I had, two flat polyps were found in my sigmoid colon. I had no idea I had these polyps because there were no signs or symptoms of them. After making the appointment for the colonoscopy, I was having second thoughts and came very close to canceling the scheduled procedure. If I had not had the colonoscopy, I would not have known I had the polyps and they could have (possibly) eventually turned into cancer. Fortunately, a biopsy was done on the polyps and no cancer was found. When I asked the doctor what I could do to prevent them in the future, he said eating more high fiber foods and less saturated fats. Here is another instance where healthy eating is so important. As a result of living a healthy lifestyle, we have a greater chance of receiving a good bill of health when we have our examinations, and a greater chance of being on the road of living a healthier life. (Note: To help reduce health care costs, consider free clinics. Also, research and inquire about free medical care and medical discounts).

Dental and Eye Examinations

Just as much as it is important to get an annual physical examination, the same holds true for dental and eye exams. A very dear friend of mine, who has the prettiest teeth, had not been to the dentist in a few years. This friend finally went when a tooth fell out and there was severe pain in another. To my friend's amazement, a deep cleaning was needed throughout the entire mouth, there was loss of bone, and there were many other dental problems. In total, all of the dental work needed was going to cost $8,500 (Eight Thousand Five Hundred Dollars).

A few years ago, I neglected to get my annual dental check-up and dental cleaning. When I went to the dentist, about a year and a half later, I just knew he was going to tell me what a good job I had been doing on my teeth. Much to my surprise, just like that of my friend's, he told me I had some bone loss around some teeth on each side of my mouth, and was recommending I see a periodontist. "No, this can't be," I thought. "I have been doing such a good job of taking care of my teeth." At least, in my mind I had.

Well, in the case of me and my friend, even though our teeth looked healthy to us, we could not see what was going on around our gums and bones. What we both had failed to do was to get our annual check-ups and cleanings. As a result, we need to visit the dentist more often than once a year until we can get back on track. That experience with the periodontist, the scraping around my bone, was no picnic, and it certainly got my attention. It had such an impact on me that I am not going to take it for granted that all is well just by what I see, but instead, I will continue to get my dental check-ups and cleanings as scheduled. I am glad to report that my last few visits have been good and I am getting great compliments during my dental exams on how I am caring for my teeth.

As part of my dental care regimen, when I drink my fruit shake, green tea and even hot cocoa, I use a (glass) straw. The use of a straw helps to reduce the amount of liquid that could otherwise have direct contact to my teeth. The straw also helps to protect the tooth enamel and reduce the amount of stains my teeth are exposed to. With the use of a straw, my teeth are more protected from the acids and other substances from the liquids that could otherwise cause possible tooth damage.

I would also like to mention that it is never a good idea to use your teeth as tools. For example, your teeth should never be used to open cans or to help tear open bags. You could cause damage, crack, or even break a tooth (or teeth), when they are used as devices in this manner. You should only use your teeth for what they were designed for, and that's to chew your food.

In addition to the importance of visits to the dentist, the other thing this experience helped me to realize was that when the bad bacteria gather around the gums and on the inside of the mouth, it seeps into the body, and can go throughout the bloodstream. As a result, this may cause other health problems, some of which could be severe. When your mouth is healthy, it helps to keep your body healthy. The simplest and the best thing to do is to get those regular check-ups and follow the dentists' instructions when it comes to dental hygiene. This includes brushing the teeth after every meal, or at least twice a day, flossing, using mouthwash, and making and keeping those recommended visits.

Another part of the body that I recommend getting an annual check-up for is the eyes. For the purpose of this section, I just want to emphasize the importance of getting regular eye exams. I would like to mention, however, it's always a good idea to wear ultraviolet (UV) protected sunglasses whenever your eyes are exposed to sunlight. This will offer great and much needed protection to the eyes from the sun's ultraviolet radiation. When your eyes are not protected from the sun's ultraviolet rays, your chances of developing cataracts are increased. (Note: Just because sunglasses are polarized does not mean they are UV protected). Also, take a break from the computer. Going hours at a time staring at the computer screen can put too much strain on the eyes.

Since I am not going into a lot of detail about the eye, here is another area where I would suggest doing some research. Just learning about the awesome mechanisms and functions of the eye can be an eye opener. As with the human body in general, the eye is an amazing organ. (See Appendix-A: A Few Facts About the Human Body).

After my periodontist visit, I decided to do a better job of doing everything possible to preserve and to keep my teeth. I want to do the same for my eyes, so I get them checked regularly as well. Just as with any other part of the body, I am the only body God has assigned and connected my teeth and eyes to. I am the one and only one who can best take care of them, therefore it is vital for me to have regular check-ups and to take good care of my teeth and eyes. The cost of a dental cleaning, an eye examination, and regular office visits for both, certainly beats huge medical bills for doctor visits, medications, or the possibility of having to undergo various procedures in order to save my teeth and/or eyes. I believe we should all make every effort to preserve and care for our teeth and eyes. (Note: To help reduce costs, consider dental schools and discount dental and eye care providers).

Colon Cleansing and Detoxifying

Like many of the issues when it comes to health care, there are differences of opinions as to what we should and should not do when it comes to our bodies. The issue as to whether or not we should use colon cleansers and/or detoxify our bodies is no different. There are pros and cons as to whether or not we should cleanse and/or detoxify. Well, here is my take on it. When you permit someone to come into your house to do work, you want them to come in, do a good job and leave. All the necessary parts that need to stay around, you want them to remain. Say, for instance, you are having your kitchen remodeled. You got a new stove, refrigerator, counter tops, new flooring, etc. You want all of those things to stay, but not all of the dust and debris that was accumulated. No matter how good of a job the contractors do, and no matter how much you like them or their work, there comes a point in time when you want them to leave; you want them and all of the trash they accumulated out of your house. However, you want them to leave all the things they put into your house that helped to beautify your kitchen.

Well, the same holds true about the food that goes into our bodies. We want it to go in and do what it has to do to fuel and provide nutrition to our bodies, and then leave. Just like the items the contractor installed to beautify your kitchen, the nutrients that need to stay around in your body should stay, and the left over debris needs to go. Hopefully, the foods that are in our bodies are the good ones because, just like a lousy contractor, the bad ones do more harm than good. But either way, whether it's the good or the bad food, after a certain period of time it needs to change its residence; the materials that need to relocate should *move* along! That which is no longer serving any purpose, you want it to leave your body and you don't want it hanging around too long. That's where cleansing may need to come into play and offer a little assistance with moving the bowels.

You may find, no matter how much you exercise, your stomach still bulges and that bulge and bloated feeling remains. Coupled with these feelings may also be a sense of fatigue. This all could very well be the result of impacted or built up fecal matter that's just sitting there in your large and small intestines — in your colon. If that build-up were to move on its merry way by being removed from your digestive system, you may very well be relieved from feeling bloated and fatigued, see a reduction in your stomach area, and even notice some weight loss. After all, all that matter that can have a tendency to pile up in your digestive system has to be visible somehow and somewhere, and it does carry a certain amount of weight.

Now, it is entirely up to each of us whether or not we cleanse or detoxify our bodies. But, for me and my house, there are times when a little extra help is needed to assist in the removal of that unwanted debris. It's not something I do on a regular basis; perhaps 1-3 times a year. As far as what I would suggest to use, I really have not found one product that I would say I am truly sold on. I have tried several different colon cleansers, but I am still taking applications and conducting interviews to find the ideal candidate (product) to do a good cleansing and detoxifying job. I have found, however, that a liquid fast for a day or two works pretty well for me. Sometimes my fasts consist of just water, and other times I will include water and juicing. Keep in mind, cleansing and detoxifying the body does not eliminate the need to eat healthy, to not overeat, and to exercise. Nor does it mean you should not have regular bowel movements, because you should.

Note: There is a difference between cleansing/detoxifying and taking laxatives. Personally, I prefer not to use laxatives. I would suggest doing an Internet search or going to your local library to learn more about colon cleansing and detoxifying the body. This may possibly help you to discover which method of cleansing and detoxifying of the body will work best for you, or if you would even want to do it.

Keep the Abdominals Tight!

The abdominals, located in the stomach area, sometimes referred to as abs, the core, or the powerhouse, are very key to the strength of your body. Some experts suggest doing abdominal exercises every day, while others say you should skip a day. I have done it both ways, but I think I prefer the every other day routine. However, the tightening of the abdominal area is something I have learned to do on a constant basis and throughout the day.

You should try to make a habit of tightening your abdominal area when doing any activity. You should tighten them to the extent where it feels as if you are trying to get your belly button to touch your spine. Not just when exercising, but when doing any activity. Example: When I take clothes out of the washer or dryer, I tighten my abs. As I reach to place the dishes into the cabinet or to take them out, my core muscles are tightened. Your core is the center of your body's strength. You may very well be surprised at how much extra strength your body gains just by tightening your core muscles when making even the simplest movement with your body. Furthermore, when your core is strong, it helps to strengthen your back muscles, improve your balance and your posture. So, if you are experiencing back pain, problems with your balance or with your posture, try tightening your abs/core muscles on a regular basis. Tighten them while exercising and when moving about doing your normal daily routines, and see if you don't notice a difference.

Note: Even with the tightening of the abs and exercising on a regular basis, if your goal is to reduce belly fat, there has to be a reduction in your food intake. Also eating good fats, like those found in olive oil, avocados and nuts, can help reduce the fat around the waist.

Getting Rest and Good Sleep

It is so important for the body to get rest, relaxation, and good sleep. For years now, I have made it a practice to take one day out of the week and do little or nothing and just rest and relax. I call this day, usually Saturday, my rest day. It is such a good feeling when Saturday rolls around and I just lounge. I don't work out, I don't prepare big meals, (leftovers are usually the meals for that day). I make every effort not to run around doing a lot of errands, I just rest on *ME Day*! It's a day filled with mostly nothingness. Obviously, there are some Saturdays when this is not possible, but for every opportunity that is presented to do so, I take advantage of this day of rest and relaxation. I think we all owe our bodies some time out to do nothing but to rest and relax. I have this saying – "*We have to either rest our body or our body is going to rest us – one or the other is going to happen first.*" The preference, however, is that we take control and rest our bodies, not being forced to rest because we have gotten our bodies into a position due to some sort of health problem – of having no other choice but to rest.

Snoring can sometimes be a problem for some people getting a restful sleep. If you have a problem with snoring, there are a few things a doctor may suggest.

1. If you are overweight, lose weight. The loss of weight could very well correct the problem.
2. Have surgery. Even with surgery, however, the snoring may or may not stop.
3. Have a sleep study conducted to see if you may possibly have sleep apnea.

If the sleep study determines you have sleep apnea, your doctor will probably prescribe a CPAP (Continuous Positive Airway Pressure) machine. The primary reason for sleep apnea is snoring. With sleep apnea, you may stop breathing many times while sleeping. It also disrupts your sleep and possibly that of any others who may hear you snoring. The CPAP machine enables you to continue to breathe while sleeping. There are some people who have been prescribed the CPAP machine and will not use it, but it's better to use it than to stop breathing and face the possibility of having a stroke or never waking up again. If you know that you snore, or have been told you do, please see a doctor, because it could be sleep apnea. Sleep apnea is not something to take lightly. It is a very serious condition and, if left untreated, could be a matter of life or death.

It is also very important for the body to get its sleep. Good sleep helps to rejuvenate the body. Some experts say that we should get at least eight hours of sleep. I must admit, this is one area that I struggle with. I only average about five hours of sleep a night. Then there are times when I fall asleep, but I have trouble staying asleep. I am a very light sleeper, so I have found when I use certain aids I get a better night's sleep. To help block out any noise I use earplugs. I discovered the kind made from silicone works best for me. Then to help block out any light, I use a sleep mask to place over my eyes. I have tried both the contoured and the non-contoured type. I like the contoured style best because my eyes do not rub up against the mask. With the non-contoured type, when my eyes touch the mask, more often than not, I will wake up.

I have been offered sleeping pills by doctors, but I chose not to use them. Rather than taking prescribed sleeping medication I know, at bedtime, it is best for me to turn off all the lights, get into the bed at a decent hour, and do not watch television but go straight to bed. So if you have problems sleeping, I suggest trying the following:

1. Have a scheduled time in which you go to bed, and stick to that time. Make every effort to go to bed at the same time each day and at a decent hour.

2. Take care of everything you need to do before getting into the bed, so that you won't have to get up hours later to take care of it. You can disrupt your sleep by constantly waking up, thinking about what you need to get up and do before it's actually time to get up. For example, don't get in the bed and then plan on getting up later to brush your teeth. Brush your teeth first and then get into the bed.

3. Wear a contoured sleep mask whenever you sleep.

4. Wear earplugs in your ears to help shut out any outside noise.

5. Turn off all the lights, including the light from the computer, before getting into the bed.

6. Get in the bed the way you to plan to sleep for the duration. Not across the bed or on top of the covers, where you will later on have to get up to reposition yourself, or find yourself constantly waking up thinking about doing so.

7. Drink your last liquid at least three hours before going to bed, so you can reduce your chances of having to get up, after you have fallen asleep, to use the bathroom.

8. Do not, and I repeat, do not turn the television on at bedtime. When it's time to go to bed, it's time to go to bed and not the time to watch television.

Now, I told you a good sleep is an area where I am currently experiencing some difficulty. So just like I am challenging you to do these things listed here, I am also challenging myself. I have no doubt the combination of these things will help me to sleep better at night, so let's try this challenge together.

Emotional Factors

Stress

Stress is that culprit that can negatively affect every part of your body and your life. It can affect you emotionally, physically, mentally, and even spiritually. So the solution is to get rid of those things that cause stress in your life, and to do those things to help reduce or eliminate it. As I mentioned previously, exercising is a stress reducer. Unhealthy foods can cause stress on the body as well. And, even though we may not always want to admit or accept it, there are certain people and/or relationships that make our lives stressful. As difficult as it may be, there are times when we have to sever certain relationships or at least distance ourselves, either partially or altogether from certain people. Anything or anyone that is causing stress in your life is obviously not in your best interest. I realize there are some things and some people that we may not be able to break away from completely, but from those we can, we should do it, and for others we can just learn how to keep our distance. The idea here is to take control of the stress and the stressful situation, and not allow the stress and the stressful situation to take control of you. You can still be in a stressful environment that may not be that easy to break away from, say on your job for instance, but you can still take control of the situation. Surround yourself with those things and those people who are positive. Not the negative things or the doom and gloom people. The positive things and the positive people will lift you up. They should be upbeat and they should encourage you. On the other hand, if you are not careful, the negative things and negative people will bring you right down into that doom and gloom state of mind along with them. Negative people like to have negative company and positive people like to have positive company. Don't join the group of the pity party people. Let them know that you choose not to participate in their, "Oh me oh my, how sad am I" program.

Worry, depression, lack of faith, low self-esteem, feeling as if you are nobody — nobody cares about you and you don't care for yourself — can all bring stress upon your life. After being a victim of an abusive relationship, I found myself having these exact feelings. I was as low as low could go when it came to what I thought of myself. I felt unloved. I felt as if I was ugly. I felt like there would never be another man who would even want or care for me. I had been mistreated to the point where I was truly convinced of all of these negative emotions. Some while later, as I started looking back on all of these hurting events that transpired in my life, I realized they were just attacks of the devil. I am the one who gave into his attacks that had me on such an emotional roller coaster and blinded me from seeing and knowing the true unconditional love of God. But during the time that I was going through all of this emotional pain, I was stressing myself out and did not even realize it. Until one day, while I was having one of my very own pity parties, the Lord spoke to me and said, "Everything I created is good, and I created you." Those words He spoke to me changed my life and put me into a new frame of mind about myself. I began to realize how much God loved me. I started to look at how He had blessed me over the years and how He continued to do so. As I looked at my life from a positive perspective, my overall way of thinking turned from negative to positive. And yes, some years later I was even blessed with a new husband. A husband who loves me, loves my son, and loves my whole family.

So if a failed relationship has you feeling stressed out, beating up on yourself, and feeling as if it's the end of the world, like I experienced, lift your head up, it's not the end of the world and you are somebody. Realize, just like the Lord told me, you are also a good thing created by God and He loves you unconditionally. There is life after a failed relationship, and you don't have to be stressed out about it.

The best way I have found to deal with stress is through the Word of God and through prayer. There was also a time when I was dealing with a lot of stress on my job. The Lord told me, "Increase the feeding of your spirit." I did that by reading the Bible, listening to good inspirational messages, prayer, and constantly thanking and praising the Lord. So when I was finally faced with the adverse situation at work, I can honestly say that I was not stressed out about it. Why? Because I was obedient to what the Lord told me to do; I was prepared for whatever was about to happen. No, I did not like what happened, I was even hurt by what transpired, but I was not stressed out about it. Matter of fact, other people could see the attacks that were coming against me on my job. One individual even asked me, "How can you be so calm with all of this going on around you?" I responded by saying, "It's summed up in Isaiah 26:3. The Lord keeps me in perfect peace because my mind is stayed on Him." In keeping a close relationship with the Lord, studying His Word, staying in prayer, and continuing to thank and praise Him, you will find this to be the best stress reducer and best stress eliminator. I've tried it and I know it works!

Alcohol, Drugs and Smoking

I do not know of anyone who wants to hear the cry or sound of hysteria in the voice of their mother. It was on the evening of November 7, 1991 that I experienced such from my mother. As she shouted into the phone through her obvious tears, I heard the words, "Little Rudy is dead, Little Rudy is dead." Because I was asleep at the time, I really thought I was dreaming. Well, I was not. My fifteen-year-old nephew, Rudolph, III (Little Rudy), the only son of my oldest brother, Rudolph, Jr. (Rudy), and his wife, my parent's grandson, and my niece's only brother, had been killed by a drunk driver. This fatal accident happened as my brother and his son stopped in the cold, snow and ice to help a motorist who had been stranded on a bridge. As my brother was attempting to help the stranded motorist, my young nephew was standing in the front of his dad's car. Suddenly, traveling at high speed, a car came zooming onto the bridge, hitting the back of my brother's parked car. My brother's car was then forced into movement, which in turn struck my nephew and knocked my brother onto the bridge to lay flat on his back by his car. My brother could not move at the time, but it was probably good that he couldn't. Because if he had been able to move, he would have looked down from the bridge where the incident occurred and saw the stiff body of his only son, lying 40 feet below on the ground of the expressway beneath.

My family was given the opportunity to speak during the trial of the drunk driver who caused the death of my nephew. While presenting my statement I said, "Individuals who choose to over-consume this 'poison' (alcohol) and then get out on the road, are not taking into account the possibility that they can take the life of an innocent human being. Neither are they taking into account the many lives that are affected by the death of one person." People are human beings and, no matter how popular or unpopular one may be, everyone is known and cared about by someone. That love and care may, of course, be in different degrees, but the fact remains that someone is affected in one way or another by a person's death.

Before my current marriage, as I alluded to earlier, I had been a victim of domestic violence. The behavior of my abuser was always triggered by the use of drugs, alcohol, or a combination of both. When he was not under the influence of these substances, he was really a good person. Here again, in my opinion, the users of these chemicals are not taking into consideration the harm they can bring to others or even to themselves. It's all a selfish act.

It is obvious that the abuse of drugs (illegal or prescription) and alcohol alters the brain and the behavior of its user. In addition, the abusive consumption of drugs and alcohol can cause so much damage to the user's body. Both drugs and alcohol can affect every body part, increase the aging process, and induce so many different health risks and problems.

Smoking contains another set of toxins that can harm the body. It too can affect every body part, increase the aging process, and induce so many different health risks and problems. It also leads to stickiness in the blood vessels, causing the flow of blood to have difficulty going through the body. In one day, the heart pumps thousands of gallons of blood that travels nearly 12,000 miles throughout the body. With the stickiness and clumping smoking causes in the blood vessels, it does not take much to imagine the stress and strain that is placed on the body as it tries to circulate the blood that wants (and needs) to make that daily journey of nearly 12,000 miles. The result of smoking positions the body for a possible stroke, heart attack, lung cancer and/or other critical health problems.

Secondhand smoke can also affect a non-smoker. Not too long ago, I saw a man smoking as he was holding a child who looked to be about 18 months old. That child was innocent, yet he was placed in a position where he was inhaling the smoke that his *caretaker* was puffing. It was not fair to the tender body of that young child, as he was subjected to the chemicals contained in that cigarette. My heart went out to that baby because he was under the "care" of the man who was smoking while holding him in his arms. Even though the man probably thought the baby was protected because he was holding him, the baby was not safe at all from the cigarette smoke he was forced to inhale.

I recently watched a television program where a discussion was held about thirdhand smoke. Thirdhand smoke, as described by a group of doctors on this broadcast, is when the smoke remains in the hair, the clothes and the skin of the smoker, and it can be passed on to others. In this particular instance, the mother of a young child was a smoker, but she always went outside of the house to smoke. What she did not know was when she would go back into the house, the residue from the cigarette smoke would still linger. As a result, when she holds her baby, her baby inhales those chemicals that are in her hair, clothes, and even her skin. Furthermore, even the furniture she sits on, as well as the air in the house, becomes infested with the toxins from the cigarette smoke.

Many of us have observed illnesses and even the death of someone as a result of smoking or chewing tobacco, or substance abuse. There is absolutely no pleasure in experiencing the death of a loved one, or watching someone die. There is absolutely no joy or pleasure in being abused or witnessing a life being taken away because of the use of drugs, alcohol or the smoking or chewing of tobacco.

I shared the tragedies and dangers above, not to badmouth anyone, but in the hopes that if you are a user or abuser of drugs (illegal or prescription), alcohol or tobacco, you will consider the harm you are doing to your body and possibly to others and their loved ones. The usage of these substances is not worth the long-term affect or damage they can do to your body. Whenever you get ready to use any of these substances, just think about the tragic consequences that could possibly occur as a result of your behavior and the many lives, including your own, that can be affected. There are organizations and support groups available that can help you through this if you have a desire to quit one or all of these habits/addictions.

Forgiveness

As my brother was interviewed from a hospital bed following the tragic accident that he and my nephew experienced, the news media asked him whether or not he forgave the driver who caused the death of my nephew. Rudy immediately said he forgave the man. He also had the opportunity to express publicly, by way of both the local and national media, how he had prayed to God for a son and how he was grateful for the 15 years the Lord had blessed him with "Little" Rudy. Even though the drunk driver only had to serve 18 months in prison, Rudy still forgave him. I had people tell me that they could not see how my brother could be so forgiving. Well, if I had not gone through what I went through with my domestic violence experience, I probably could not have understood it either.

As a result of being a victim of domestic violence, I had developed hatred towards my abuser. After all, why should I not hate him, since he constantly made me feel like an ugly nobody and since he had abused me both emotionally and physically, even while I was carrying our baby? My hatred was justified and forgiveness was not necessary. God and everyone else should be in agreement with me, because I had every reason under the sun to feel this way towards him because of all he had done to me. Well, at least that's what I thought and truly believed was totally right and justifiable at the time.

What made me change my way of thinking happened three years after our healthy son was born. While sitting in the front of a church, I was listening to a Christian radio broadcast. As I was about to turn the car off to go into the church, a woman was ministering. As I reached for the key to turn off the ignition, she said, "If you are holding unforgiveness and harboring bitterness in your heart, you are not giving God any room to bless you. Harboring bitterness and unforgiveness is like a cup that has been filled to its brim. It's so full that nothing else can get into it. So how can God bless you when you have a heart filled with bitterness and unforgiveness? Just like there isn't any more room in that cup filled to the brim, you are not giving God any room to bless you." WOW, her words hit me so hard. I knew then that I needed to repent and ask for forgiveness for harboring such ill feelings towards another person. Once I did that, I felt like a ton of bricks had been lifted off of me. It was also at that time that I vowed to never allow myself to be possessed by such a destructive and ungodly emotion as hatred towards another person. A few years after hearing that broadcast, my abuser asked for my forgiveness, and I sincerely forgave him.

When we don't forgive, we do more harm to ourselves than we do to any one else. It's like carrying a poison around in our bodies. And, as with any other poison, unforgiveness can do more harm than good to our bodies and/or to our lives.

In Mark 11:22-24 it reads: *"...Have faith in God. For verily I say unto you, That whosoever shall say unto this mountain, Be thou removed, and be thou cast into the sea; and shall not doubt in his heart, but shall believe that those things which he saith shall come to pass; he shall have whatsoever he saith. Therefore I say unto you, What things soever ye desire, when ye pray, believe that ye receive them, and ye shall have them."* Many times when we read this passage of Scripture, we stop right there. We claim that God will answer our prayers if we just believe it, when we pray it, and have no doubt in our hearts that what we are asking is going to happen. That is true, but the answering of our prayers comes with a condition. God will do His part in answering our prayers for those things we have the faith to believe, but we have to do our part as well. In addition to having faith in God, having the belief, and having no doubt in our hearts that what we pray will come to pass, we must forgive. As we read the next two Scriptures, Mark 11:25-26, we see where Jesus goes on to say, *"And when ye stand praying, forgive, if ye have ought against any: that your Father also which is in heaven may forgive you your trespasses. But if ye do not forgive, neither will your Father which is in heaven forgive your trespasses."* Forgive, and you will be forgiven.

Forgiveness is not an option but a necessity; it's a command. In addition, it helps to relieve stress and eliminate those possible health issues caused by stress. There are too many people who hold grudges, refuse to let go of a hurt from the past, and refuse to forgive. When one holds a grudge, that grudge becomes a barrier and one of the functions of a barrier is to block. If you are holding grudges, being bitter or harboring unforgiveness, you position yourself to block your blessings and it is not worth the possible consequences. Refusing to forgive is a sin, it goes against the Word of God, and it hurts you more than anyone else. Forgiveness does not only include forgiving others, but forgiving yourself as well. Forgive those who have wronged you in any kind of way (no matter what the circumstances are) and forgive yourself for the mistakes, errors or even harm you may have brought upon or done to yourself. Don't keep beating yourself up from past sins. Forgive yourself and move on. Furthermore, once you have confessed your sin(s), repented (turned away from them), forgiven another (or others), and/or forgiven yourself, be sure to ask God for forgiveness and receive it. I John 1:9 states, "*If we confess our sins, he is faithful and just to forgive us our sins, and to cleanse us from all unrighteousness.*" Speaking from experience, you will feel so much better when you forgive another, (or others), forgive yourself, ask God for forgiveness, and receive His forgiveness.

Chapter 12

In Conclusion: Make Plans to Be in Your Future

It was March 19, 2000 around 9:15 AM when once again I received two different telephone calls with the same horrific news. The first call came in from my sister-in-law, and the second one from my daddy. As Daddy was talking to Phil, I had already begun to scream, shout and cry out, "No...No...No!" As I lay stretched out on the floor, beating into it with disbelief, I could hear the loud screams of my mother coming through the telephone. We had just been notified that my brother Rudy's private plane had crashed and he was instantly killed. When the plane crashed, it went up in flames, and Rudy's body was burned beyond recognition. "No, not my brother, this just can't be true," I thought. But it was true. At a young age of 49, it was Rudy. Rudy was older than me by two years, and he and I were the two eldest children of five. I, as well as the rest of my family, still miss him so much, but I have no doubt in my mind that he and his son (my nephew, Little Rudy) are reunited, as they have both physically left this earth and gone home to be with the Lord.

Even though the tears and the pain have subsided, and since my brother and his son (my nephew) had a personal relationship with Jesus Christ and are spending eternity with Him, there is still rarely a day that goes by that I do not think about one or both of them. When special family events come up or family decisions need to be made, I often think about the things my brother would say or do. My brother really enjoyed flying his plane. I know how much the plane meant to him, and the passion he had for flying, but I can't help but wonder the *what ifs*.

- *What if* I had tried to get my brother to think about the affect it would have on his loved ones if something happened to him in his plane?
- *What if* he had never thought about the possibility of something happening to him until I brought it to his attention?
- *What if* he had taken into consideration the overall affect a tragedy in his plane would create, and then decided to stop flying altogether?

- *What if,* as a result of these discussions, my brother would still be alive today?

I know I will never know the answers to all of these *what ifs* as well as other questions that I have. It may possibly sound as if I am beating myself up with the *what ifs*, but I'm really not. However, I can't deny that I have had my share of the *what if* thoughts and moments. There is nothing that can be said or done by me or anyone else to bring my brother or nephew back to this earth. I can no longer communicate with them face-to-face as I had done in the past. I can't ask my brother the *what if* questions, but this is just another reason why I am so adamant, determined, and feel so strongly about communicating and reaching out to as many people as I possibly can about living healthy. And how I hope and pray, since they are still alive and while they still have breath in their bodies, they will decide to incorporate the things it takes to live a longer and healthier life.

At much younger ages than witnessed in the past, too many people are being stricken with sicknesses, diseases, severe health problems and even premature death, as a result of unhealthy lifestyles, poor eating habits, and lack of physical activity. By changing over to a healthy lifestyle, people have a better chance of extending the duration of their life and feeling good as they complete its journey. I am not talking about a temporary *diet*, or a *diet* at all for that matter, but committing to living a healthy lifestyle for the rest of one's life.

As I started out saying at the beginning of this book, it is my sincere desire to see everyone healthy. I want to do what I can to help others do all they can to take better care of their bodies. I want to do what I can to help those who may otherwise end up asking themselves the *what if* questions.

- *What if* I had only started eating right? Perhaps I would not be faced with this illness.
- *What if* I had only started exercising? I would not be having these aches and pains.
- *What if* I had only shared with my loved one the importance of proper eating and exercising? Maybe they would still be alive today.

The list of *what ifs* could go on and on. The good news is, however, the *what ifs* don't have to be *what ifs* in this instance. The *what ifs* could very well become *what*.

- This is *what* I am going to do to live a healthier lifestyle.

- This is *what* I am going to do to be around longer for my family.

- This is *what* I am going to do to take better care of myself.

- This is *what* I am going to do to see my child/children grow up.

- This is *what* I am going to do so my grandkids can know me as their grandparent.

- This is *what* I am going to do to make plans to be in my future.

One may ask, "How can you make plans to be in your future?" Well, we make plans for everything else in life.

- We make plans for special events.

- We make plans to go to work day after day.

- We make plans to take our cars in for service.

- We make plans to take vacation.

- We make plans for retirement.

- We even make plans for death. We make wills and take out insurance policies. Some people go as far as selecting and purchasing their caskets, burial plots and even the clothes they want to be buried in.

We make plans for this, that and the other, so why shouldn't we make plans to be in our future? When we make plans for special events, for going to work, for taking our cars in for service, for taking a vacation, for retirement, death, etc., we always make some sort of advanced preparation. Some preparations are greater than others, but the fact remains that preparations are made for anything we plan. Just as we make plans and preparations for everything else in our lives, we should certainly want to make plans to be in our future. The primary way in which we can do this is to make the preparations now by taking good care of our bodies. The healthier we are, the better our chances become of living longer and healthier lives. On the other hand, the unhealthier we are, the slimmer our chances become of living a long and healthy life.

If you are having difficulty with incorporating a healthy lifestyle, think about your loved ones who care and love you:

- Think about what affect it would have on their lives if you were not in their futures.

- Or, you are so sick that you wouldn't be any good for them, yourself or any one else.

- Also, think about how an unhealthy body can inhibit or prohibit you from doing the things God has called you to do.

Many of us think that the things we see happen to other people could not possibly happen to us, so we continue on with our unhealthy ways. But the truth of the matter is that they can. Anything we see happen to someone else could very well happen to us. Whether it's as the result of substance abuse, unhealthy habits, poor food choices or lack of exercise, none of us are exempt from the consequences associated with living an unhealthy lifestyle. But there are those steps (as mentioned in this book) that we can take to reduce our chances of becoming another negative statistic.

Certainly, I realize that none of us will live forever on this earth, but we don't have to rush our departure either. And that's exactly what we do when we choose to neglect and abuse our bodies. We abuse our bodies when we subject them to unhealthy things, when we choose to deliberately consume unhealthy foods, and when we do absolutely no form of exercise...that's abuse. But it does not have to be that way. The question in the title of this book asks, *Are You Helping Your Body Live?* After incorporating into your life the suggestions I have outlined in this book, the answer to that question would be an absolute **YES!**

Throughout life, we are constantly faced with having to make choices, and the choices we make have consequences. Matter of fact, we are faced with making choices all throughout each day. Renewing your mind about taking positive steps towards the healthy things you can do for your body, taking control of your eating habits, and doing some type of physical activity are all choices. Committing to a lifetime of a healthy lifestyle is a choice. You either do it, or you don't. But as with any other choices we make, an unhealthy lifestyle has consequences and so does a healthy lifestyle. If you have not done so already, it is my prayer that you will make the decision to do those things that have a healthy impact on your body, to make healthy food choices, and choose exercise as an important part of your life. If you are doing those healthy things for your body, are eating healthy and nutritious foods, and have incorporated physical activity (exercising) into your life, I pray that you will continue to do so for the rest of your life.

Speaking of prayer, as previously mentioned, prayer has played a major role in helping me through my healthy lifestyle journey. Like I have already stated, our lives are full of choices, and as for me, I choose to believe in the power of prayer. I have no problem admitting this healthy way of life has its challenges at times, but prayer has helped me and continues to help me to overcome those challenges. My personal relationship with the Lord, my prayer time and devotional time with Him, have really made a big difference in my life. At the end of this book, I have included a list of confessions that have been helpful to me. I have shared it with others who have found it to be uplifting and encouraging to them as well, and I pray that you will find it to be the same for you. (See Appendix-B: True Confessions).

I realize there are thousands of health-related materials on the market, and you should continue to educate yourself in this area. I am constantly learning as much as I possibly can when it comes to living healthy. There are now so many different health shows on television, as well as websites that we can learn from. Perhaps some of them may not be as creditable as others, but there are some that are worth looking into. I have many of my favorite websites listed at the end of this book, and I highly encourage you to visit them.

If you really think about what so many of the other healthy living advocates and I have in common, the key to living a healthy lifestyle is making healthy food choices, exercise and taking supplements. However, as previously mentioned, if you find you are having difficulty in these areas, please pray about it. And even if you are not having difficulty, pray that you can maintain such a lifestyle. With all these components coming together — prayer, healthy choices and exercising — you may find they do wonders for your life even more than you can ever imagine.

As I conclude, it is truly my heart's sincere desire that you spend your future living a healthy, long, and great quality of life with those you love and care about, and who love and care about you. Please choose to live a healthy lifestyle!

It's Your Assigned Body!

As you entered into this world on

your day of birth,

your body became your residence

for your entire time on this earth.

To have and to hold 'til death stops its heart, you've been

assigned to take loving care of each and every part.

So as plans are made for different

events that are days or years ahead of you,

please be sure to include the future of your

health and of your body too!

♥

Appendix A

A Few Facts About the Human Body

Here are just a few facts about the body the average human being is carrying around:

- It has 206 bones (350 at birth)

- It has more than 600 muscles

- It has about 76 organs

- The average number of cells in the human body is between 75 and 100 trillion

- 300 million cells in the human body die and are replaced (most of them) every minute

- The heart pumps an estimate of 8,000 gallons of blood that travels nearly 12,000 miles per day

- The heart beats around 35 million times per year

- There are 45 miles of nerves in the skin of a human being

- There are 60,000 miles of blood vessels in the human body
- Your body is 70 percent water
- The human brain is about 85 percent water
- There are 10 million nerve cells in your brain
- There are over 100 million light sensitive cells in the retina (a part of the eye)

As you research different facts about the human body, you may find the above numbers vary, depending on who reported them, but the variations are not that diverse. However, the fact remains that the numerous amounts of the various mechanisms that God has designed to operate the human body are so awesome! There is so much about this gift of life that we often take for granted, but it is so amazing to think about all of the many functions, some even in the trillions, that are going on throughout the body as long as there's breath in it. Each and every body part knows exactly what its function is and faithfully carries out its duties on a daily basis. When the body, and its parts, is properly taken care of and is in good operating condition, it can deliver its best performance in the way in which God created and designed it to function.

God loved you (and He still does) so much that He gave you this gift of life. Let Him, and your body, know how much you love and appreciate it by taking very good care of it. Love yourself, not in a way of conceit, but in a way of expressing to God your appreciation for your gift of life. As with anything you love, you make every effort to demonstrate that love and how much you care. Well, your body deserves that same sort of love, care and treatment. Remember, your actions should certainly speak louder than your words.

Appendix B

True Confessions

Confess these Scriptures and the prayer out loud with boldness. Say them over and over again so that they can get deep into your heart. God is true to His Word and He gets pleasure out of us reminding Him of what He has said in His Word. He is faithful to perform what His Word says. Note: ( ) is the Scripture reference for each confession.

- I confess with my mouth the Lord Jesus Christ and believe in my heart that God raised Jesus from the dead. (Romans 10:9)
- I am a sinner, but because of Jesus Christ, I am saved by grace. (Ephesians 2:5)
- Jesus is my Lord and Savior. (Philippians 2:11)
- I am more than a conqueror through Christ Jesus my Lord. (Romans 8:37)
- No weapon formed against me shall prosper. (Isaiah 54:17)
- I have the Greater One living on the inside of me, therefore I have overcome any obstacles that may try to come my way. (1 John 4:4)

- I cast all of my cares upon the Lord because He cares for me. (1 Peter 5:7)
- God has not given me the spirit of fear. (2 Timothy 1:7)
- I am the righteousness of God through Christ Jesus. (2 Corinthians 5:21)
- I put my trust in God, therefore I will not fear what man can do to me. (Psalm 56:11)
- I have perfect peace because my mind is stayed on the Lord. (Isaiah 26:3)
- No evil shall come upon me, neither shall it come near my house. (Psalm 91:10)
- I can go to Jesus whenever I am feeling weary or heavy burdened and He gives me rest. (Matthew 11:28)
- When I delight myself in the Lord, He gives me the desires of my heart. (Psalm 37:4)
- I have the mind of Christ. (Philippians 2:5)
- God loves me! (John 3:16)

<u>A Prayer of Thanksgiving</u>: I thank You, Lord, for saving me. Thank You, Lord, for always leading me to triumph in Christ Jesus. I thank You for all that You have done, all that You're doing, and all that You are going to do in my life. Thank You, Lord, for being You and for who You are to me. I thank You for Jesus and I thank You for Your Holy Spirit. I thank You for Your living Word. I thank You that I can confess Your Word over my life, and it shall not return unto You empty but it shall accomplish that which is pleasing to You. Thank You for loving

me so much. I love You, Lord...In the name of Jesus I pray...Amen!

References, Resources & Suggested Websites

Note: I am not promoting the sale of any products that may be associated with any of these websites. Please use these links as a starter point to lead to other related topics you may want to research. I highly recommend doing further research on these topics. Remember, the more you learn, the more you know. The more you know, the more you can do what it takes to live a longer, healthier and better quality of life.

1. *Walking as an Exercise*:
   http://www.medicinenet.com/walking/article.htm

2. *High Cholesterol*:
   http://www.emedicinehealth.com/high_cholesterol/article_em.htm

3. *Medication Side Effects*:
   http://healthtools.aarp.org/drug-directory/drugs-B

4. *Obese Children*:
    http://www.themoneytimes.com/featured/20100211/
    obese-children-risk-dying-prematurelystudy-id-
    10100101.html

5. *Healthy Foods*:
    http://www.fruitsandveggiesmatter.gov/benefits/inde
    x.html

6. *Junk Foods*:
    http://www.medicinenet.com/script/main/art.
    asp?articlekey=56170

7. *Fibroid Tumors*:
    http://womenshealth.about.com/od/fibroidtumors/
    a/knowabtfibroids_2.htm

8. *Torn Cartilage/Meniscus*:
    http://www.arthroscopy.com/sp05005.htm

9. *Osteopenia*:
    http://www.webmd.com/osteoporosis/tc/osteopenia-
    overview

10. *Menopause*: http://www.menopause.org/

11. *Insomnia*: http://en.wikipedia.org/wiki/Insomnia

12. *Antioxidants*:
    http://www.healthcastle.com/antioxidant.shtml

13. *Free Radicals*:
     http://longevity.about.com/od/researchandmedicine/
     p/age_radicals.htm

14. *Human Cells*:
     http://www.madsci.org/posts/archives/2001-
     02/981770369.An.r.html

15. *Glutathione*:
     http://www.youtube.com/watch?v=Eh2PYQBICWs

16. *Immune System*:
     http://www3.niaid.nih.gov/topics/immuneSystem/

17. *Kidney Disease*:
     http://www.kidney.org/atoz/content/potassium.cfm

18. *Spices as Antioxidants*:
     http://spices.suite101.com/article.cfm/healthy_
     cooking_with_spices

19. *Dangers of Artificial Sweeteners*:
     http://www.healthiertalk.com/artificial- sweeteners-
     are-they-safe-0747

20. *Dangers of Sugar*:
     http://www.therawdiet.com/dangers-of-sugars.html

21. *Cancer Loves Sugar*
     http://www.alternativehealth.co.nz/cancer/sugar.htm

22. **Different Names for Sugar**:
http://www.dietriffic.com/2009/03/26/names-for-sugar/

23. **Dangers of MSG**:
http://www.naturalnews.com/020550.html
and
http://www.becomehealthynow.com/article/dietbad/32/2/

24. **Different Names for MSG**:
http://www.truthinlabeling.org/ hiddensources.html

25. **MSG/Cancer & Other Health Problems:**
http://www.msgtruth.org/cancer.htm

26. **Processed Foods:**
http://bodyecology.com/07/10/18/hidden_dangers_of_processed_foods.php

27. **Eating Disorders**:
http://en.wikipedia.org/wiki/Eating_disorders

28. **Food Labels**:
http://www.fda.gov/Food/LabelingNutrition/ConsumerInformation/ucm078889.htm

29. **Trans Fat:**
http://www.bing.com/health/article/mayo-125000/Trans-fat-is-double-trouble-for-your-heart-health?q=trans+fats&FORM=FFF

30. *Coconut Benefits*: http://www.coconut-info.com/

31. *Cocoa Powder*:
http://www.astrologyzine.com/healthy-chocolate.shtml

32. *Juicing*: http://www.juicing-for-health.com/juicing-lessons.html

33. *Bragg Products*: http://www.bragg.com

34. *Olive Oil Benefits*:
http://www.whfoods.com/genpage.php?tname=
foodspice&dbid=132

35. *The Healthy Benefits of Eating Nuts:*
http://www.sixwise.com/newsletters/ 05/06/29/
if_you_are_nuts_about_
health_try_the_top_6_healthiest_nuts.htm

36. *Soaking Nuts*: http://www.raw-food-living.com/soaking-nuts.html

37. *Body Inflammation*:
http://www.bodyecology.com/06/12/28/inflammatio
n_ cause_of_disease_how_to_prevent.php

38. *Obesity*: http://www.cdc.gov/obesity/index.html

39. **Calorie Track:**
    http://www.mayoclinic.com/health/calories/WT0001
    1
    and
    http://www.caloriescount.com/free_FoodCalculator.a
    spx

40. **Body Mass Index (BMI):**
    http://www.aarp.org/health/healthyliving/
    bmi_calculator/

41. **Wheat & Gluten:**
    http://www.glutensecret.com/wheatintolerance.html

42. **Salt/Sodium Intake:**
    http://www.mayoclinic.com/health/sodium/NU0028
    4

43. **Benefits of Exercise:** http://www.webmd.com/fitness-
    exercise/benefits-of-exercise

44. **Atrophy of the Muscles:**
    http://health.kosmix.com/topic/Atrophy_Of_The_
    Muscles?p=hl&as=yhoo&ac=478

45. **Types of Exercise:**
    http://www.becomehealthynow.com/category/
    exercisetypes/

46.　**Target Rate Zone**:
http://www.americanheart.org/presenter.jhtml?
identifier=4736

47.　**Children & Exercise**:
http://kidshealth.org/parent/nutrition_fit/
fitness/exercise.html

48.　**Hand Washing**:
http://www.mayoclinic.com/health/hand-
washing/HQ00407

49.　**Snow Removal:**
http://abcnews.go.com/Health/HeartFailureNews/he
art-attack-risk-shoveling-
snow/story?id=9812385&page=1

50.　**Household Products**:
http://www.cbn.com/media/player/index.aspx?s=/
vod/SUE149_KathyLoidolt_061009_WS&search=h
ousehold%20cleaners&p=1&parent=0&subnav=false
and
http://www.cbn.com/700club/guests/bios/Kathy_Loi
dolt061009.aspx

51.　**Food Addictions**:
http://www.allaboutlifechallenges.org/food-
addiction.htm

52.　**Importance of Drinking Water**:
http://www.everythingatkins.net/water.html

53. **Plastic Bottles Leaching Chemicals**:
    http://www.cbc.ca/consumer/story/
    2006/12/21/bottle-study.html

54. **Nutritional Supplements**:
    http://www.drlwilson.com/Articles/why%20
    take%20supplements.htm

55. **Turmeric (Spice) Benefits**: http://autoimmunedisease
    suite101.com/article.cfm/turmeric

56. **Vitamin D**:
    http://www.cbn.com/cbnnews/healthscience/2008/Ja
    nuary/ Vitamin-D-Cancers-Natural-Enemy-/
    and
     http://www.litalee.com/shopexd.asp?id=392
    and
    http://health.usnews.com/usnews/health/articles/070
    608/0608health.vitamind_2.htm

57. **Grapefruit & Medication**:
    http://www.webmd.com/hypertension-high-
    blood-pressure/guide/grapefruit-juice-and-medication

58. **Dental Care**: http://www.wikihow.com/Take-Care-
    of-Your-Teeth

59. **The Human Eye**:
    http://www.pasadenaeye.com/faq/faq15/faq15_text.h
    tml

60. ***Colon Cleansing/Detox***:
    http://www.articlesbase.com/non-fiction-articles/colon-cleansing-detox-benefits-194982.html

61. ***Sleep Deprivation***:
    http://www.betterhealth.vic.gov.au/BHCV2/bhcarticl es. nsf/pages/Sleep_ deprivation?OpenDocument

62. ***Sleep Apnea:*** http://sleepapnea.org/

63. ***Stress***: http://www.stress.org/

64. ***The Effects of Alcohol***:
    http://www.drugfree.org/Portal/drug_guide/Alcohol

65. ***The Effects of Illegal Drugs, Alcohol & Smoking***:
    http://www.brainsource.com/brain_on_drugs.htm
    and
    http://www.yesican.gov/drugfree/drugeffects.html

66. ***The Effects of Smoking***:
    http://www.cdc.gov/tobacco/data_statistics/fact_ sheets/health_effects/effects_ cig_smoking/

67. ***Help For Drinking Alcohol***:
    http://www.drugfree.org/Intervention/ GettingHelp/How_to_Cut_Down_on_ My_Drinking

68. ***Help To Stop Use of Illegal Drug Usage & Alcohol***:
    http://www.addict-help.com/findtreatment.asp

69. ***Help To Stop Smoking***:

    http://www.smokefree.gov/Default.aspx

Favorite and/or Other Informative Websites

1. http://cbn.com/health

2. http://www.knowthecause.com/ (Website/Television host believes many chronic diseases, including cancer, could in fact be — or be caused by — fungus and/or mold. The host contends that fungus can be found in corn, corn products, peanuts and peanut products and should be avoided. Please visit this web site, or watch the television show, and learn more about this interesting concept).

3. http://www.doctoroz.com/

4. http://saveourbones.com/

5. http://www.thedoctorstv.com/

6. http://www.yourhealthtv.com/

7. http://www.cspinet.org

8. http://www.usda.gov

9. http://www.thedailygreen.com/

10. http://www.fda.gov/default.htm

11. http://www.corsinet.com/trivia/h-triv.html

12. http://www.ama-assn.org/

13. http://www.biblegateway.com

Personal Health Assessment Websites

1. http://www.lifesupplemented.org/scorecard.htm

2. http://www.northwesternmutual.com/learning-center/the-longevity-game.aspx

3. http://www.realage.com

About The Author

RUNAE L. GARY is the second child of five born to Elder Rudolph, Sr. and Mattie M. Perry in Cleveland, Ohio. Runae attended the Cleveland Public School System. She holds a Bachelor of Arts degree from Kent State University, Kent, Ohio and a Master of Business Administration degree from Samford University, Birmingham, Alabama. She is also a 2008 graduate of RHEMA Bible Training Center in Broken Arrow, Oklahoma.

Runae has an extensive background and work history in Human Resources Management, Equal Employment Opportunity, Employment Discrimination, and the various laws regarding these areas. Runae also enjoys teaching as well as sharing and spreading the Word of God. Although she has a number of years working in positions related to human resources, her sincere passion is in the health and wellness area. Having a true desire to help people learn how to live longer and healthier lives, she has helped many people with their various health challenges.

In addition to *Are You Helping Your Body Live? — Effective Ways for a Healthier Lifestyle*, Runae is also the author of *Surviving the Troubled Waters — Scriptures for Meditation,* available in the New International Version (NIV) and the King James version.

Runae is the wife of Phillip Gary, Jr., the mother of Paul Gabriel Favors, Jr., (LaTasha) and the stepmother of Phillip Michael Gary.

LaVergne, TN USA
13 December 2010
208462LV00002BA/4/P